I
Ca
dba Moonridge
Integrative Cancer Connection

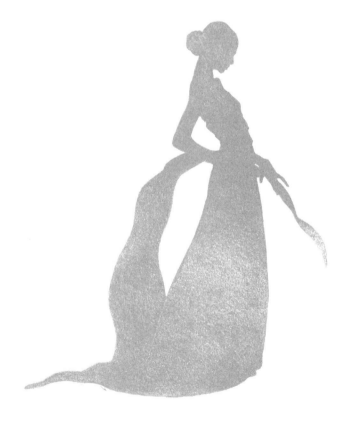

Dreamwalk

*A Survivor's Journey
Through Breast Cancer*

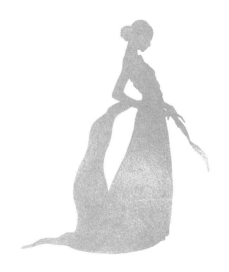

Dreamwalk

*A Survivor's Journey
Through Breast Cancer*

Rachael Clearwater

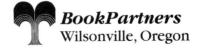

BookPartners
Wilsonville, Oregon

Cover Art by Kara Richardson

Cover Design by Aimee Genter

Copyright 2001 by Rachael Clearwater

All Rights Reserved
Printed in the United States
Library of Congress Catalog 2001 131205
ISBN 1-581-51-103-5

BookPartners

P.O.Box 922
Wilsonville, Oregon 97070

Dedication

To my husband, Stan,
for his constant encouragement through
my healing process
and during the writing of my story,
My love, always.

Table of Contents

Preface ....*xi*

Chapter 1   Prelude *1*

Chapter 2   Dreamwalk *17*

Chapter 3   Flowers, Friends and Aspirations *33*

Chapter 4   The Hands of an Angel *47*

Chapter 5   Challenges—Living with a Time Bomb...........*55*

Chapter 6   The Light..*79*

Chapter 7   20/20 Hindsight *95*

Chapter 8   Helpful Suggestions *107*

Epilogue *109*

Preface

Thousands of American women are finding themselves caught in the grip of a relentless killer, a disease which has taken on the proportions of an epidemic. The words *Breast Cancer* strike fear into our hearts, because the statistics are all too familiar: One in Eight. Every year, one in eight women over the age of forty is given the frightening diagnosis that will alter the course of her life forever. This woman is not just a cold statistic. She is a mother, a wife, a lover, a friend, a sister, a daughter —the list goes on and on. Her life has meaning and value. Suddenly her world is ripped apart, and she finds herself thrown into rapidly moving currents of unfamiliar waters. Rocks gouge and bruise her body, and icy water fills her lungs. The experience is almost indescribable.

In November of 1994, I became the "One in Eight." After the living nightmare faded, I gave considerable thought to what I could have done differently had I been better informed.

This book is intended to tell my story and share information which may be of value to other women facing a breast cancer diagnosis and the ensuing surgical procedures. This narrative is also a journey to the "light at the end of the tunnel."

Although most of the emphasis in these pages rests with my mastectomy experience, much of the information may be helpful to all breast cancer patients as well as to their families and friends.

Not everyone opts for immediate reconstructive surgery, and some of us, for whatever reasons, will enter the alien world of chests rather than breasts. At best it is a harrowing experience, but with the right information, several potential stumbling blocks can be avoided.

In retrospect, I would have done a few things differently. However, I do take full responsibility for my personal pitfalls. For that reason, I have purposely omitted naming any of my doctors.

A cancer diagnosis is something for which no one can really be prepared, but despite the turmoil and terror that rages, decisions must be made relatively quickly and should be made with the knowledge that the results are somewhat permanent. Unfortunately, assertiveness is often difficult to achieve in the face of total chaos.

Letting the professionals call the shots is not only more comfortable but seems totally natural. Sometimes their decisions are correct, but when they screw up (and they do!), YOU wear the scars and YOU pay the price. Sometimes that price is high—you pay with YOUR life.

I hope the following narrative may lighten the load for anyone traveling the dark, treacherous path that breast cancer so fiendishly maps out for its victims. If even one woman is spared a single negative experience on her journey to wellness, this book will have served its purpose.

Rachael Clearwater

Acknowledgments

My gratitude and appreciation to:

Barbara Smith, Carolyn Clapp, and Linda Sullivan
for helping me with this story.

Peggy Wood for giving me a typewriter.

Judy Allen, Deepak Chopra, Norman Cousins,
Louise Hay, and Bernie Siegel for enabling me
to reshape my thinking.

My dear friends Evalyn Guernsey and
Penny McLaughlin for providing positive feedback.

And most of all Virginia Jones for giving me the courage to
keep going when I was ready to give up and throw it all away.

and

To All Who Touched My Life So Lovingly.

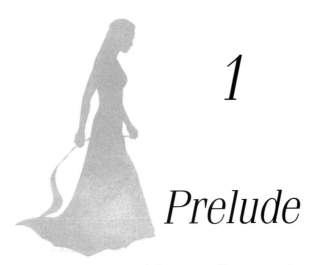

1

Prelude

"Sometime in your life, you will go on a journey.
It will be the longest journey you have ever taken.
It is the journey to find yourself."

— Katherine Sharp

I think I always knew I'd make this journey someday. I don't know how I knew; it's beyond my understanding. Maybe my soul knew.

The day remains burned indelibly on my mind. I was sixteen that summer. When I close my eyes and think back, I can still catch the scent of the lumber mills—slash and sawdust burning away in the huge blackened incinerators at the edge of Yreka. We didn't call it pollution then. It was the smell of our town, of our industry. We lived with that.

I had just placed my copy of Leon Uris' *Mila 18* face down on the coffee table and was more or less unconsciously running my hand over the surface of my chest when suddenly, without warning, my life changed forever. There it was—under my fingertips— a small lump no bigger than the eraser at the end of a pencil. How could this be? I was only a teenager!

For what seemed like the longest time, I sat frozen in space and time on our mint-green sofa, unable to think. When the words finally tumbled to the surface of my mind, they repeated over and over in my head—a nightmarish refrain of fear and terror.

This must be breast cancer. I remembered it from one of my health classes. One of the warning signs of cancer: *A lump or thickening in the breast or elsewhere.* Beyond that, my knowledge was relatively sketchy. What I did know was that I simply couldn't deal with it now; the thought of being diagnosed with breast cancer was altogether too overwhelming. So I made a conscious decision. No one must know what I had found, not even my mother. For the next two years, my days were spent vacillating between raw anxiety and total denial. Every so often, I would feel for the lump, hoping it had somehow magically disappeared. It never had.

In the fall of 1963, while lying on my bed in the dorm at Chico State College, I routinely felt for the pea-sized lump and collided instead with something the size of an olive. Dear God, this was it! My worst fears were becoming reality. The lump had grown, and my life would be over. At the very least, I would be permanently maimed and no one would marry me, in which case I might just as well get it over with and cash it in now.

For some reason, I decided to tell a friend in the dorm. She immediately hauled me off to the housemother, a sweet, elderly woman who was also a retired registered nurse. Mrs. A. assured me that, given my age, the mass was almost certain to be benign. She also insisted that I consult a physician. I was mortified, but complied. The doctor did a routine breast examination and promptly sent me home to Yreka for a biopsy, the only available diagnostic tool at the time.

The wretched lump was finally sliced from my body, and I was advised that I had a condition known as cystic breast disease. In no way did that condition imply a predisposition to cancer, or so I was told. The relief was overwhelming. The following week, I returned to school with a one-inch scar across my left breast. But the saga was far from over.

During the next few years a series of various sizes of

palpable lumps appeared in both breasts, mostly before my periods. Often they vanished as unobtrusively as they appeared. My anxiety levels varied as much as the silent comings and goings of these unwelcome intruders.

In 1965, I decided to pursue a dance career and moved to Los Angeles to study ballet. My apartment was two blocks from the Panaieff Ballet Center on Beverly and La Brea, and I thought I had wandered into Camelot. Dance became my life, as I spent my days traveling from studio to studio, determined to follow the urgings of my spirit. An occasional lump would rear its ugly head, but my mind was on other, happier things. These bumps were harmless cysts, and most of them went away. I just danced them away.

Being in Los Angeles gave me a sense of belonging, of fitting in. The studios and audition halls were filled with young hopefuls, sharing my dreams of ballet companies and movie contracts. Yreka had been an idyllic place to grow up, a place free of the stresses of city life. But I had often found myself feeling somewhat out of place—a distant relative on the outside looking in. My friends took naturally to all of our high school activities, but try as I would, I couldn't muster an interest in rock n' roll or football. To add to my misery, I had discovered that I was definitely a late bloomer. All around me, people were falling in love while I sat on the sidelines wondering what it was all about and why it wasn't happening to me. Los Angeles proved to be a healing balm. My life was finally beginning to come together.

Eventually I decided it was time for a short trip home. I would be the dancer from "Big Time L.A." in the small-town dance studio. My teacher lived on the Rogue River a few miles south of Grants Pass, Oregon. Her name was Daryle Holt, and she was wonderfully eccentric, with her bleached-blonde hair and her spike heels from Henry Waters in Portland. More than my teacher, she was my Auntie Mame. I would sit entranced as she recounted exciting tales of days spent on the road, dancing in theaters and night clubs up and down the West Coast. She had even done a short tour with the Ballet Russe de Monte Carlo. Her home was always open to her students, and to me it had often been a refuge. The next few days would be no exception. After a visit with my family in Yreka, I headed for Rogue River.

The afternoon sun beat down on our backs as we sat on the banks of the river, dipping our feet in the warm, green water. Daryle lit a Pall Mall (straight) and looked at me over a half-empty bottle of Bud. "I'm taking Goldie up to Portland to audition for a club job. Are you interested in going?" She squinted at me in the bright sun.

Goldie was my best friend in the studio. No one could match her humor, and whenever we were together, we always laughed to the point of tears. I thought for a moment. My plan had been to spend at least two years in Los Angeles studying and auditioning, but I had made no close friendships, and the idea of working as a dancer, collecting a paycheck, was not without appeal.

"What about my classes with Panaieff?" I asked.

"It's up to you, but Portland has some good teachers, and you could still take daily classes. The experience would probably be good for you."

"Where's the job?"

"There's a club in Portland called Gracie Hansen's Roaring Twenties. They have a six-girl line. The pay isn't anything to write home about, but it's enough to live on, and you and Goldie could split expenses."

The words tripped out of my mouth, "Yeah, I'd like to do it. Sounds like fun."

Auditions in Los Angeles had been packed full of polished dancers, most of whom had already worked and acquired their union cards. I had gone to a few cattle calls but hadn't had any luck. Maybe this would be a place to start—that is, if I could get in. After all my classes with Panaieff, I'd feel like a total fool if Goldie were hired and I was left in the dust. Oh well, too late to turn back. So we piled into Daryle's powder-blue Cadillac and hit the road for Portland.

The Roaring Twenties Room was beyond grandiose. The stage was raised for the performances and lowered to floor level for dancing between shows. The curtain was red velvet, and a huge mirrored ball hung from the ceiling, rotating to send a shower of sparkling light in every direction. The men's toilet was a festive attraction, and Gracie Hansen treated the patrons to a nightly tour between shows. The facility sported a statue of Fidel Castro, and when the patrons whizzed in his mouth, his eyes lit up. We were duly impressed.

The choreographer lined everyone up and gave us the once-over. This definitely wouldn't classify as a cattle call. Only about ten girls had answered the ad, and several of those were obviously not dancers. After the usual combinations and a series of pirouettes, Goldie and I were both asked to stay. Rehearsals would start the following morning.

We rented a tacky room at the Park Avenue Hotel and shopped at Newberry's for falsies, false eyelashes, and our version of stage makeup. We must have been a sight, with our bright-blue eye shadow smeared generously from our eyelashes to the bottom of our eyebrows. No one corrected us until several months later when Daryle and a few friends came to Portland and dropped by to see the show. She wasted no time informing us that we looked like a couple of hookers and gave us a crash course in how to use makeup in the right places to accentuate and bring out our "natural beauty."

The show at the Roaring Twenties consisted of a band, a chorus line, two fully clothed showgirls, a banjo act, a male trio and Gracie Hansen, a Sophie Tucker-type woman who was reputed to have been a madam in the logging town of Morton, Washington. I had my doubts, but it made a good story. The dancers had four production numbers, and the smoke in the club was so thick we could hardly breathe, but we were in show business. This was big stuff.

The vocal trio was exceptionally good, especially the bass. His name was Stan, and he was preparing to leave for New

York the minute the show closed. Occasionally he would join us in the hotel coffee shop between shows, and I eventually learned that he was thirty-seven years old and that his wife had died, leaving him with a son and a daughter who lived in the country with their grandmother during the week.

In some strange way, something about this stocky, unpretentious man intrigued me—something that transcended my respect for his talent. I found myself thinking about him, wanting to know much more than he had chosen to tell me. What was he really made of, this sandy-haired bass in his well-worn desert boots and tweed sports jackets?

Finally, Gracie heard that Goldie and I were walking home after work to save cab fare and asked Stan to be our chauffeur. Sweet serendipity! By now we had upgraded our living conditions and were staying in a downtown hotel with a small heated pool on the roof. Often the three of us would go for a late-night swim and relax in the sauna after the show. Soon we were swimming nearly every night and had developed a nocturnal ritual of sorts. One Saturday night Goldie bowed out and turned in early, exhausted from a long and rigorous week. She had been attending cosmetology school in addition to working at the Roaring Twenties.

Stan and I decided to go swimming anyway and found ourselves sitting at the edge of the pool talking non-stop until daybreak. He told me of his plans to study in New York with Metropolitan Opera buffo, Salvatore Baccaloni. As he talked about his love of opera, he became at once completely charged with enthusiasm. His absolute lust for music created an atmosphere of hypnotic energy. I had never given opera a second thought, yet as he spoke of *Tosca* and *La Boheme,* I felt myself being drawn in to the point of thinking about hopping a plane to New York to see this magic for myself. Finally we dressed and continued our conversation in the downstairs coffee shop.

Over tea and bagels, we decided to drive to the beach. I'd never seen the Oregon coast, and the first sight of the vast expanse of ocean in its spectacular setting of soaring trees and rugged rocks was spellbinding. We parked the car and walked for a while on the beach, eventually settling on a damp, weathered log deposited on the white sand by the endless ocean tides. As we sat there together looking silently at the distant, sun-streaked horizon, I finally admitted to myself that I was beginning to feel much more than a casual attraction for this "older man." But the moment of revelation brought with it an overwhelming sense of sadness, because I knew in my soul that in a few short weeks he would be gone forever. His heart was already three thousand miles away.

Then, as we got up to walk to the car, something completely unexpected happened. He took my hand. It was a small gesture, nothing earthshaking, but at that moment I could feel that the chemistry was there, and its strange power was traveling full circle. There on the beach, at that precise moment, the die was forever cast. I knew I would go to New York; I just didn't know how.

Our show closed, and he was gone. Misery set in like a bad case of acne. Even the glamour of working in the show did nothing to alleviate my emptiness. I couldn't eat. I couldn't sleep. Something simply had to give before I perished in the drama of a broken heart.

A gig at Izzy's Supper Club in Vancouver, B.C. finally solved my dilemma. One of the girls in the show had an apartment in Greenwich Village and had decided to remain on the West Coast to be married, so she flew back to New York with me to collect her belongings, and I moved into her place. The apartment was a five-flight-walk-up, cold-water flat with a toilet off the kitchen and a small bathtub adjacent to the kitchen sink. The plumbing was economically connected. Every time I took a bath, I found myself cleaning scraps of food from the tub before I could run the water. The building had no lock on the main front door—ergo no security. I could hear footsteps stomping on the roof well into the early morning hours, which I assumed were signs of ongoing drug deals. The place was less than safe and very primitive, but to me it was *West Side Story* all the way.

Stan had an apartment in midtown Manhattan, and we started seeing each other the minute I hit the Big Apple. He took me to a little cafe at the edge of the Rockefeller Center ice rink, and we sipped chilled May wine as we talked about music and theater in the balmy June breeze. Auditions, he said, were a necessity. I had only planned as far as lessons, but he had already performed with two small opera companies and felt sure that I would be able to plug in somewhere. He seemed to have more faith in me than I had in myself. I loved being in New York, but I questioned the possibility of finding work there as a dancer. This was the center of everything: talent was pouring out of every door, and the competition was fierce. In any event, I was much more wrapped up in romance than in the idea of advancing my career.

Life was good. My days were spent taking classes, studying with some of the teachers I had only read about: Luigi, Salvadore Juarez, Jaime Rogers—they were all right there. The streets of Manhattan were filled with young hopefuls toting dance bags, propelled by their dreams of being invited to join a ballet company or landing a Broadway show.

Evenings were even better. Stan and I were together constantly, soaking up the flavor of this bustling, never-sleeping city, savoring ethnic food and cheap wine in the intimate atmosphere of quaint little sidewalk cafes in the Village.

A few weeks had passed when I read in *Variety* and *Backstage* that Lou Walters was holding auditions for a replacement in the line at E.M. Loew's famed Latin Quarter. I decided to muster up my courage and check it out. Couldn't hurt—no one knew me. The audition was unusually short. After a series of pirouettes and a parade across the stage, two girls were asked to stay. To my utter astonishment, I had been chosen. Mr. Walters was up in years, and I could only surmise that he didn't see too well, because the other girl was wearing braces on her teeth and sported a smile resembling the grille of a '52 Buick.

We were sent backstage to see Ernie, the stage manager,

a rotund gentleman with black hair and a pencil-thin mustache. Ernie looked at us and rolled his eyes. There was no opening at this time, he said. A bit miffed, I inquired whether he would at least take our names and phone numbers in case one of the dancers dropped dead in the near future. Unknowingly, I had made a smart move. A few days later, a girl decided to leave the show, and I was hired.

My dream was coming true. The Latin Quarter featured some relatively well-known headliners, and when we weren't dressing or dancing, we were free to sit in the wings and watch the celebrities do their stuff. Sid Caesar was my all-time favorite. I couldn't get enough of his genius. To think I was sitting not more than fifty feet away, breathing his air! All that talent. I was star struck.

For the next few years, I enjoyed the limelight and the razzle-dazzle of New York. When the show at the Quarter closed, I was hired almost immediately at the Copa where some of the headliners were Dionne Warwick, Tony Bennett and The Temptations. I was definitely in great company.

One night before the show, I heard that a scout from the William Morris Agency was in the audience. This could be my big chance to advance my career. During the first production number, I was really outdoing myself, selling up a storm, when I suddenly slipped on a grape (the patrons ate right at stage level) and slid on my hindquarters across the edge of the stage and halfway under a table. The audience howled, but my two minutes in the spotlight did nothing to get me discovered.

Finally in 1968, Stan asked me to marry him. I didn't have to think twice. We hopped the subway to the New York City Hall with two of our friends and made it legal. Somehow Earl Wilson's column got wind of the event and printed that I was a "nudenik cutie." Our costumes were relatively brief, but we were far from nude. Furious and sputtering, I demanded a retraction, which was promised, but of course never happened. Naturally, one of my mother's friends spotted my name in the Atlanta paper and sent a clipping to my family. That little bit of embarrassment was the sum total of my New York notoriety.

During those storybook days in New York, I don't remember having found a single lump. Maybe I was just too happy to notice, I don't know. My health was the farthest thing from my thoughts. But the New York chapter of our lives was nearing its final page.

Stan's two children, David and Margaret, had been living with their maternal grandmother in Oregon for some time. Now that we were married, we felt we should be a family. Reluctantly, we said good-bye to New York and headed back to the West Coast.

My requirements for an immediate income were pressing, and I enlisted the services of an employment agency. The owner thumbed through a card file and made a quick telephone call. She didn't actually tell me where she was sending me, muttering instead something about calling on overdue accounts. As I pulled up in front of the address she had given me, I was immediately taken aback. This place was a collection agency. I'd heard about their business tactics and the thought of working in such a place did nothing to quiet my nerves. But I desperately needed a job. My mind raced as I envisioned knocking on doors with a weapon tucked into my belt demanding overdue payments from frightened people.

The owner of the company was a cherubic little man who immediately decided to ask me something which would give him some insight as to whether I had any assertiveness skills. "What makes you think you can collect bills?"

Fresh from the New York rat race, I wasn't short on chutzpa. "What makes you think I can't?"

It worked.

"When can you start?" he asked with a grin on his face.

"Tomorrow," I quipped back.

He sat me next to his top collector and told me that if I could do what she did, I'd make good money. I listened, and I caught on. The job was the pits, but the commissions were good. Day after day I sat at a desk arguing with people about money. Days ran into months, and months became years. Time after time, the lumps in my breasts came and went—no more bothersome than a hangnail— weaving their way in and out of my body and my life like a familiar, haunting refrain.

It took me a long time to realize that I hated sitting at a desk, and I hated the confrontational nature of my job. Alcohol had become a permanent fixture in my life. A little glass of Chablis after work, and I was lulled into euphoria. Soon I was putting it away by the bottles. No-Doz and aspirin were getting me up, and alcohol was knocking me out.

By 1986, I'd had enough of my go-nowhere, dead-end lifestyle. Funny how life can drag along day after day, until one day you finally know when you've had enough, My boss had died, and things were changing. I gave two weeks' notice and walked out into the sunlight. Within six months I had dried out, and I've been stone sober ever since. Before long, life took on meaning again. The birds were singing, and the flowers were blooming. I was a born-again *person*. There was an awakening and a sense of heightened awareness that kept me floating ten feet above the ground. I was experiencing a knowing of my natural essence. Surprise! My spirit was intact!

The next job opportunity that came along was different from anything I had ever imagined. I will always believe that God himself led me to children who needed special education. I loved my job as an educational assistant from the onset. The kids were magic. Despite their erratic behaviors and disabilities, handicapped children have a wonderful honesty about them. They're just "out there" — all up front. For the first time in seventeen years, I felt as though I was making a contribution, putting something back into the world. What a contrast to the unhappy world of lawsuits and levies.

The school system provided an excellent benefit package, and since I hadn't been to a doctor for several years, I decided it was probably time. By then, mammography had come on the scene, and I opted to schedule an appointment. After all, I was in my forties and had a history of lumpiness. For me, the procedure was surprisingly painless, though I had heard tales of woe from women who were considerably better endowed than I. The technician flattened each breast and told me not to breathe for a few seconds while she took an X-ray. No big deal.

Or so I thought. Two or three days later, I received a message at work that a mass of 1.5 centimeters had been detected at "11:00 o'clock" on my left breast, exactly where my cyst had been removed in 1963. It appeared "worrisome," they mumbled. My heart pounded so loudly I could hear it like a kettle drum in my ears. Mild unrest was replaced by stark terror.

My imagination ran mad. Aunt Ruby, one of my favorite relatives, had lost her left breast several years earlier, and I knew the surgeons had removed not only the breast, but several lymph nodes and massive amounts of muscle tissue. She was fine for a few years until cancer showed up in her colon. I had watched in horror as she valiantly battled the monster disease year after year, never knowing when to expect the descent of the final curtain. Was my life taking an unexpected turn down the same dark road?

I telephoned my doctor the minute I arrived home from work and was reassured that eighty percent of "these things" are totally benign. Being the insecure soul that I am, I immediately focused on the other, not so fortunate, twenty percent. My mind raced for a few days until a decision was made to schedule an ultrasound. To the best of my understanding, it was a painless procedure by which sound waves were utilized to project an image of the inner breast onto a screen. Such a test could distinguish between fluid-filled cysts and solid tumor mass.

As the dreaded day approached, I became increasingly anxious. Sleep became elusive. I found myself lying awake playing and replaying variations of the worst-case scenario. Between panic attacks, I would attempt to dwell on the possibility that I would fall into the fortunate, healthy eighty percent, those lucky souls who would go home with a giant weight lifted from their shoulders, those who would be able to go on with their lives unscathed and unchanged.

All too quickly, it was time to go. Although the day itself was warm and balmy, an icy phantom wind swept through my entire body and took up residence, refusing to leave. Try as I would, I couldn't shake it. My stomach was quivering out of control. For some reason, I didn't take Stan along with me. He had been very concerned about my state of mind and had offered to go, but somehow I felt that if I fell apart, I needed to do it alone. I checked into the area marked "Radiation/Ultrasound" and was given the familiar directions, "Everything off to the waist." Now I would be even colder.

The technician was a young woman, probably in her late twenties or early thirties. She applied some cold (of course) gel to my chest and ran a metal contrivance to and fro, all the while watching the images on a screen and making notations. I attempted to convince her to divulge the dark secrets of the mystical imaging, but she tactfully advised me that the results would be sent to my doctor. Another eternal wait. Anyone who would wish to slow the passage of time should try waiting for the results of a questionable breast exam. The hours just don't come any longer.

Finally my doctor's nurse called me and said that the ultrasound reflected several fluid-filled cysts and that I should have an annual mammogram. The roller coaster had temporarily come to a shaky halt. Relief flooded over me like a soft, balmy breeze. Life resumed for another year.

In 1991 I had another mammogram. Well trained, I took off my clothes above my waist, looking on as the technician took several slides of my left breast. I got dressed again from the waist up and was sent on my way. Once again, I waited. I waited.

This time the call came directly from my doctor. This couldn't be good. My mind raced. Surely it was a bad sign! Why would she take time from her busy schedule to call me personally? Unless, of course, she was the bearer of some dreadful news.

My good doctor was very apologetic. It seemed my

X-rays from the previous year had been misplaced and could not be compared with the new ones. She felt we should "err on the safe side" and aspirate. I wanted no part of it. By then I had the distinct feeling that maybe doctors and procedures just weren't for me.

"Every time I go to the doctor, they find something wrong. Obviously, the logical solution is never to go to the doctor." I was exasperated and it showed.

She was very patient. "I realize it feels that way. I understand what you're trying to tell me, but we need to work together to get this resolved."

I thought then and still feel that I have the nicest doctor on the planet. We scheduled an appointment with a surgeon across town.

This physician's office building was a real study in depression. It was a big, dark, foreboding building called *Comprehensive Cancer Center.* Probably, I mused, it was owned by an affluent group of morticians who wanted to scare the hell out of everyone and hustle up some extra business from those poor souls who'd drop dead from sheer fright. *This too shall pass,* I assured myself silently.

If my initial impression was one of fear and apprehension, this doctor made up for it. He instantly won me over with his caring, soft-spoken gentleness. After discussing my history and reading my X-rays, he decided against aspirating. He said that "given the amount of scar tissue from your previous biopsy, this is normal topography for your breast."

Those were words I have since grown to regret taking at face value, but I was ecstatic at that moment. I thanked him and left the black box of a building feeling totally healthy and a bit smug. Strange how the words of a medical professional have the ability to alter our perceptions in an instant. I thought about my general practitioner. Perhaps she was overly cautious? Perhaps she had a colleague who was sued for malpractice, so she sent her patients for unnecessary procedures in order to play it safe?

The next time I was in her office, I recall telling her confidently that I had no family history (Aunt Ruby was related by marriage) and wasn't really at risk. I still remember her words. "*We're all at risk.*" I didn't really think so. More than twelve percent of women are diagnosed with breast cancer, *and I didn't really think so?* What arrogance on my part.

The year 1992 brought another routine mammogram and a welcome call from my doctor advising me that everything had stabilized. I was fine. Life was good. I was so relaxed and confident that I coasted until 1994. I was on my own dream walk.

Then the bomb hit ground zero.

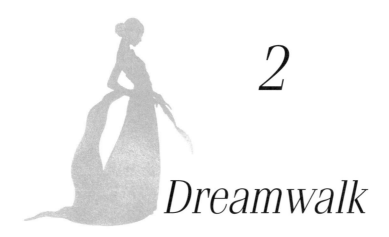

2

Dreamwalk

*"Your fear of death is but the trembling of
the shepherd when he stands before the king
whose hand is to be laid upon him in honour."*

—Kahlil Gibran

October of 1994 was an unusually beautiful month. The leaves were more brilliant than ever, and the neighborhoods were filled with the festive air of ghosts and little orange pumpkin lights. Stan and I were jogging every night, and I felt as strong and healthy as ever, both physically and spiritually. The only down side of my life was that my ninety-one-year-old mother had come to live with us and was showing alarming signs of oncoming dementia. She and I had always had a wonderful, close relationship, and watching this sweet, gentle woman gradually lose her mind was like burying her an inch at a time. But that was my only major stress factor, and I felt I could handle it better than most people, considering my experience of working with physically and mentally disabled children. Little did I know what was lying in wait just a bit down the road.

I scheduled a mammogram and joked with the technician about how I always required several retakes because of my residual scar tissue. She was out of the room for what seemed like a long time. Finally she opened the door and said flatly,

"You were right. We need another picture. The radiologist doesn't think it's scar tissue."

She flattened my left breast again and disappeared from the room with the plates. I was beginning to get edgy. She returned and told me I could get dressed.

"The radiologist is going to recommend a biopsy, so be prepared," she warned me, without a trace of sensitivity in her voice. I remember saying something about not having time to be sick because I had a ninety-one-year-old mother to take care of.

"Better to find out now than later," she responded coldly. I drove myself home with her words echoing in my head. It all seemed surreal.

When I arrived home, the installer from Sears was just leaving. We had ordered a new storm door, and I was anxious to see it. As I walked through the kitchen, hoping for one bright spot in a day that wasn't shaping up very well, I noticed that the new door hadn't been installed. Stan started to explain something about a dent in the one the man had brought. We would have to wait for another one to be sent from the warehouse. Nerves tight, fear choking me, this rather insignificant, trivial incident of a flawed screen door was the proverbial straw that broke the camel's back. I let fly with an inexcusable line of profanity— shouting about my pain and blaming it on Sears.

Stan was understandably embarrassed and tried to smooth things over.

"I'm sorry! They think I have cancer," I blurted out and stormed upstairs. Because Stan didn't follow me and ask for details, I immediately decided he was insensitive and probably didn't give a damn. Nothing else was going right. My husband might as well be indifferent to my probable date with the Grim Reaper. I hadn't read *Men Are From Mars, Women Are From Venus*. After twenty-seven years I still expected him to handle everything the way I do, with lots of dialogue, bare-faced emotion and frustrated passion. I just hadn't learned yet! Later we talked, and although he listened intently, he didn't respond. I didn't know how to read his silence. A couple of weeks later he told me that words failed him. He just didn't think it could happen to me.

My doctor was out of town for the next few days. Another endless wait. We finally connected, and she provided me with the unwelcome particulars. The mass that had shown up on the mammogram was two centimeters in size and appeared on the X-ray as a "starburst." I later learned that the so-called "starburst" was the actual spread of the cancer—*infiltrating ductal carcinoma.* She attempted to soothe away my terror, but it had me in its choke hold.

"It may not be anything evil. It may just be scar tissue. Scar tissue is sometimes mistaken for a tumor mass."

What else could she say? She tried.

She suggested an appointment with the same surgeon I had seen three years earlier and I readily acquiesced. Subconsciously, I viewed him as a ray of hope in the dark. After all, this man had sent me away happy before. I even waited two weeks for him to return from a vacation. Maybe he would make it all okay.

This time I asked Stan to go with me. The doctor did a breast exam and was unable to detect a palpable mass. Maybe it was gone. Maybe they were totally wrong. Maybe God had taken it away. I got dressed and waited to see my X-rays. We sat in a cheerful little room with plush sofas, and I thumbed through leaflets relating to breast surgery. After a few minutes, the nurse poked her head in the door and said we could come out and talk with the doctor.

In his office, my X-rays—back-lit— were hanging on a wall, and for the first time I was able to see the nefarious starburst. The doctor pointed to it with his finger and explained that it appeared "worrisome." There was that bloody euphemism again. What was worrisome to him was beginning to scare the hell out of me. We returned to the cheerful little room, which by now had taken on the aspect of a cold and confining jail.

The doctor was of the opinion that we should "go after it." He would do a wire insertion followed by an excisional biopsy. He began to explain a technique whereby a wire is inserted into the exact center of the mass with the help of a computer image. This enables the surgeon to locate the precise spot when he's doing his cutting. I was scheduled for the two procedures on November 8th, a "Day That Would Live in Infamy."

Life took on the quality of a dream sequence. Everyone at work tried to help me to remain positive, especially David, one of the assistants in our classroom. Everyone felt sure it would prove to be benign. I mentioned the prospect of a mastectomy, and David assured me that they weren't doing much of that any more. Stan didn't talk much, but I felt his support. Everyone in our church, especially the members of our choir, surrounded me with love and concern.

As the days passed, I felt as though someone else was living in my skin, living my life. I was frightened, but not really panic stricken, as I had expected. Only once can I remember actually crying. Lying in bed one evening, a wave of reality suddenly hit me. I sobbed a few times, and it was over. The dream continued. Maybe that reaction is part of being in a state of shock or protective denial. I don't know. The days passed relatively quickly. Somehow I knew the grim reality of my situation.

November 8th rolled around. The following is an entry from my journal:

Today I checked into the hospital in the early morning hours. A technician and his assistant performed a "wire insertion" in my breast. It was awful. I found myself lying face-down on a table with my breast hanging through a huge hole, while two people worked underneath me, ramming a wire with a hooked end into my flesh. I felt violated and helpless. Tears streamed down my face as I tried to breathe deeply and cry in silence. My doctor had explained the procedure to me, but no one had warned me I'd be lying face-down, unable to see anything.

This was just the beginning.

Probably I reacted differently than other women, due to the fact that I had an unfortunate sexual experience with an older boy at an early age. Even years later, an assault on the more private areas of my body triggered unpleasant memories. This procedure felt like a definite assault. The only comic relief to the situation was the size of the hole in the table. It was as big as a pie pan, and I was thankful that I wasn't having a wire stabbed into a size 44D. At least if I lost a breast, they wouldn't have to cart it off to pathology on a hand truck. Later I reflected on my lack of sensitivity as I thought how much more difficult everything must be for women with large breasts.

When the procedure was completed, I was sent to a room to wait for surgery. The ugly wire protruded through my dippy hospital gown. Stan stayed with me for a while and then left to check on Mama. My "cut time" was set for eleven o'clock in the morning, but it was three hours past the scheduled time before I was finally wheeled into pre-op. My anesthesiologist came in and offered me two options. I could have a general anesthetic, in which case I would be longer in recovery, or I could opt for twilight sleep (such a beautiful name) and go home earlier. Thinking about my mother, I chose the latter because it promised a shorter recovery time.

I saw an intern strolling by, chomping away at a hamburger. How could he be doing something as casual as stuffing his face when I was about to go under the knife? It reminded me of a cartoon I'd seen of a policeman filling out his paperwork while he was sitting on a homicide victim. Life was going on merrily for the rest of the world while mine was caught in a crazy, dream-like web.

Finally my surgeon appeared at my side and we talked briefly. He told me that he would remove the lump and the surrounding tissue. I would have the results from the lab in two days. Somehow his blue gown gave me a sense of security.

Shortly after he left, I was taken to surgery. Because of the twilight sleep, I was able to hear everything that was being said, so I eventually heard someone ask for more tissue.

I remember thinking or verbalizing an obscenity. Even in a semi-conscious state, I knew the implications. As they wheeled me back into my room, I saw Stan standing in the doorway. Drowsily, I gave him a thumbs down.

My surgeon came into my room and discussed the size of my tumor. He admitted that it was slightly bigger than they had expected. The conversation was marked by the obvious omission of the C-word.

"So you found cancer," I challenged him, as I looked squarely into his eyes.

He side-stepped. He still didn't say the word. He replied that the mass was a malignant tumor, but still avoided the word "cancer." He took my hand, and suddenly I felt sorry for him. What must this part of his job do to him, having to tell people that their lives are threatened by a dreaded disease? That the prognosis is not rosy? That their lives may be coming to a painful end?

I sat for a moment trying to maintain my composure. My body felt unsteady, and I was having difficulty processing what was really happening. Finally I spoke, but the words didn't seem to be coming from my mouth—they were just suddenly in the air.

"Will I have to have chemotherapy?"

I had always feared chemo. I had pitied its poor, ghost-like victims—those poor souls without hair, their eyes sunken deeply into their skulls, in what I had imagined was probably fear, coupled with a degree of hopeless resignation.

He responded that I should come to his office the following day. We would discuss treatment options at that time, after the pathology report was in. I began to shake uncontrollably. My teeth were chattering. Stan later told me that I had looked like a hundred-year-old woman while I sat hunched over on my hospital bed that day.

One of the nurses came to my side and tried to comfort me by telling me that there was hope. Her heart was in the right place, but hope wasn't what I wanted. *What every cancer patient wants is the assurance of a cure, assurance that there will be NO recurrence*—something that no one can give us.

On the way home in the car, my anger finally kicked in. This was bullcrap. It was the kind of thing that happened to smokers, drinkers, meat-eaters and mean people. Suddenly I felt like some sort of loser. Stan reminded me that Aunt Ruby had lost a breast to cancer and asked me if I considered *her* a loser. His words shut me up but did nothing to dissipate my anger. The shaking continued.

When we arrived home, I had a pressing need to go off somewhere alone and indulge myself. I wanted to cry or shout or stomp my feet or throw something against the wall. But Mama was waiting to see me. She understood little of what was happening at any given moment. I needed time to think before I gave her any explanation, not wanting to add more unhappiness to her already sad and frightened, shrinking little world. Maybe it was a blessing that she wouldn't really understand everything. In her right mind she would have taken it all very hard. I was her only child, born to her late in life, and we were very close. She had been the most wonderful mother anyone could ever ask for. Almost on a daily basis she had always told me that I was the best thing that had ever happened to her. Now that I was caring for her, she thanked me profusely for every little thing I did for her. I loved her beyond measure.

We sat down at the dinner table. Mama always inquired about my day, and this would be no exception.

"Did you have a nice day?" she asked. The humorous aspect of her question brought a welcome touch of levity, and a slight smile broke across my face as I thought of various unspoken answers. I had enjoyed this day about as much as the barnyard goose enjoys Christmas dinner!

"It was okay. I'm a little tired. Think I'll turn in early." Obviously she thought I had just returned from work. This was not the time to tell her anything, I decided. Perhaps later—much later. I dragged my weary body upstairs, undressed in the welcome comfort of our bedroom, and went to bed.

Despite my exhaustion, I couldn't sleep, so I set about the task of updating a few of my closest friends about my "condition." I had promised I would call. Barbara, an old dance buddy of mine from the Roaring Twenties days, had been waiting and praying. She had always been my Rock of Gibraltar.

"What did you find out?" she urged.

I didn't wait on ceremony and blurted out, "It's malignant and tomorrow I go back to discuss my options."

Dead silence on the other end. Finally a faint, almost shaky voice—not typical of my friend, Barbara.

"That blows my mind. I can't believe this is happening to you." I sensed the unshed tears in her voice.

I couldn't really grasp the verdict myself. I knew it was real, yet somehow I felt as though the experience belonged to someone else. We talked for a long while. I know that some people avoid dialogue about their condition, especially about a frightening diagnosis and a less than certain future. I've never understood how they manage to do that. Talking things through has always been a necessity for me. Speaking openly with Barbara that night and listening to her loving responses and concerned comments gave me a sense of inner peace. We were two old friends who had shared life's ups and downs so often along the way. Our friendship went back over thirty years. The compassion in her voice was beginning to dilute my feeling of isolation. I was grateful to have such a solid, good friend with whom to share my sorrow.

After the initial shock had worn off, Barbara started doing what she does best — one of the things I love in her. She began radiating strength, even power. We talked about my upcoming birthday and the fact that I could use a warm bulky robe and something with which to pad my bra after surgery. And I could use lots of prayers. I needn't have mentioned that. God was the central focus in Barbara's life. Little wonder she was such a sturdy rock.

Before I could make my next call, the phone rang. It was Penny, my other local soul mate. She too was a former dancer from the Roaring Twenties. Just as Barbara was my rock, Penny was my down comforter—a sensitive, intuitive soul whose feelings for others run steady and deep. Often she would waltz through the front door for a visit and take her place next to Mama, stroking her hand and talking with her as though they were the only two people in the world. Penny would be a true blessing in the days ahead.

As I recounted the day's events to my friend, I understood her mounting alarm. Penny had lost both her father and her half-brother to colon cancer. She had once remarked that she considered the cancer question for her to be not *whether,* but *when.* She had felt sure that my biopsy would be negative, considering that there was no history of cancer in my immediate family. We talked until drowsiness began to overtake me.

I replaced the phone in the cradle and was suddenly overcome by complete exhaustion. Sleep embraced me like a warm blanket on a cold day. As I drifted off, the thought occurred to me that never having to wake up might be pretty nice. Even in a state of semi-sleep, I knew that the next day wouldn't show up on the "gratitude list" of my diary. Tomorrow was bound to be an ordeal, especially when the nirvana effect of the drugs had worn off.

As Stan and I drove to the doctor's office, I pondered the time off work, wondered about my accrued sick leave and envisioned myself completely bald. I touched my hair. There's something about hair, a woman's "crowning glory"—or something like that. I could end up bare and bald. I shuddered at the thought. Time, time! Only time will tell. My thoughts raced on. Mama. What if I couldn't beat this thing? Stan couldn't possibly care for her alone. This whole experience must be magnified beyond belief for women with young children to raise. Enough!

The moment we pulled into the parking lot, the shaking reappeared in the pit of my stomach. The time had come to "discuss my options," as the surgeon had so delicately put it. I had been expecting a lumpectomy and maybe some chemo or radiation. From everything I had read or been told, the survival rate was about the same for mastectomy and lumpectomy procedures.

Seated across from my doctor, I searched his face for a hidden message. Nothing. It was business as usual. What was "usual?" How many times in the course of his work week did he have to face a frightened, shaking patient, perhaps carefully choosing words to lighten the load of a black verdict—maybe even pronouncing the death sentence? I wondered.

He explained quietly that I had something called infiltrating ductal carcinoma, the most common type of breast cancer. In a soft monotone, he recommended a modified radical mastectomy as my best choice.

I froze. Nothing could have really prepared me for that statement. This man was actually telling me that I should have my left breast removed...cut, whacked off. The dream sequence was evolving into a nightmare. Had I heard him correctly?

"Remove the entire breast?" my voice almost squeaked.

"You could opt for a lumpectomy. It's your body. But I'd advise a mastectomy." His voice was toneless. I tried to take a deep breath to clear away the elephant that sat on my chest, but it wouldn't budge. I felt as if I were suffocating, and I tried to think. This man was a doctor, a medical professional. He must know what would be best. *I didn't even ask why.* He went on to explain that the breast and surrounding lymph nodes would be removed. If the node dissection proved positive, the survival rate up to fifteen years was 50 percent. Negative nodes increased the figure to 75 percent. My God! This meant that death definitely hovered within the realm of possibility. If the nodes tested positive, I could just as easily die as not.

The dream walk I was experiencing must have been some sort of shock absorber, because waves of fear rushed in and out of my consciousness, never staying for long. The constant fear came later. I heard my next words but I couldn't feel my mouth moving.

"Just get it over with. Schedule it as soon as possible."

To this day I don't really know what happened in that office and why I didn't ask for more information. Maybe I'd felt intimidated. I'd never called doctors by their first names, and I had always accepted wasting long periods of my time waiting for a few moments of theirs. Here I was being told that I should have one of my body parts removed, and I felt uncomfortable questioning the judge and the verdict. How absolutely absurd!

We sat for a few moments in an ominous silence while I struggled to process what I had just heard. Finally the doctor broke the spell. "We need to decide whether you want reconstructive surgery performed at the time of the mastectomy."

That suddenly sounded good. "Might as well do it all at once and get it over with." I managed to sound cavalier and mask my true feelings.

"I'll have to line up a plastic surgeon. It will take a little longer. Also, I need to explain to you that the recovery is longer," he stated.

"How much longer?" I wanted to know.

"It can take up to seven weeks."

"How long without reconstructive?"

"Three to five weeks. Sometimes less."

"Just schedule the mastectomy. I'm not even sure I have that much sick leave, and I don't know whether my insurance would cover plastic surgery."

Stan spoke up. "If it isn't covered, we'll just pay for it. Don't we have money in savings?" This was and continues to be one of the things I have always loved about my husband. He wouldn't have hesitated for one second if it had meant spending our last dime. It was only money.

The main thing I couldn't deal with was the idea of having to wait longer for the surgery. Lining up a plastic surgeon would take more time. I wanted the ordeal behind me—over, done with as soon as possible. We scheduled the surgery for the following Tuesday, three days before my forty-ninth birthday.

The ride home seemed endless, wrapped in silence as

thick as a London fog. Stan finally spoke. "You're a rock. I don't know how you do it."

"Do what?" I questioned.

"Stay so cool," he replied. "If this were happening to me, I'd be yelling at the top of my lungs and climbing the walls." His hands gripped the wheel.

"That's a nice compliment. I guess I just don't know how to react. None of it seems real. It's almost like an out-of-body experience. The doctor just told me that in six days I'll actually be disfigured, and I can't take it all in. It's like it's happening to someone else." I stared out the window not seeing anything.

The moment we arrived at home, I called Barbara again.

"Well? What did you find out?" she asked anxiously.

"That I'm losing the breast."

"WHAT??!"

"That's what the doctor advised. I could have reconstructive surgery at the same time, but the recovery takes longer, and I'm not sure my insurance would cover it."

Barbara had recently undergone breast-implant surgery and was extremely pleased with the results. She offered to call her plastic surgeon and see what he had to say. I told her I'd appreciate any additional information she could obtain.

A day or so later she called me. "My doctor recommended that you have a plastic surgeon do the closing if you're considering having reconstructive surgery in the future."

That bit of information proved to be something I ignored and later regretted. Here again, I wasn't comfortable asking my surgeon to bring someone else in just to close the incision. What if he were insulted? What if he thought I didn't trust him to do a good job? There's that "doctor-on-the-pedestal" again! I was more concerned about hurting his feelings than looking after my interests, my future.

For the next few days, I avoided looking at my left breast. I remember reading a story many years ago about a woman who had lost her leg to cancer. From the time her surgery was scheduled, she never shaved the leg she was about to lose. Now

I understood her completely. Identifying with the breast in any way would make its impending loss harder to face.

One of my high school friends, Ruthie, was a nurse in Bellingham, Washington, so I decided to pick her brain and inquire about the surgery and exactly what to expect during my time in the the recovery room. Perhaps I could ease my anxieties if I had some idea of what would be going on around me. She suggested that I "get educated" and take an active role in the decision making from here on out. She recommended two excellent books, *Dr. Susan Love's Breast Book*, and *Breast Cancer, The Complete Guide*, by Yasher Hirshaut and Peter Pressman. Both books are extremely informative, and I would recommend them as required reading for any woman facing breast surgery for cancer. I read both books from cover to cover, storing every word in my memory bank. I would need it all.

One fact I hadn't known was that in the event of a recurrence, barring a miracle (and I do believe in miracles), cancer can never be cured. It can only sometimes be put into remission. That thought terrified me. Apparently one isn't afforded a second chance to defeat this horrendous disease. One wrong decision can prove fatal. Also, breast cancer, unlike many other forms of cancer, can pop up twenty years down the road, although the odds of having been cured increase with each year of cancer-free survival. Pretty scary stuff.

During that time, some of my perceptions changed noticeably. The thought that we are really not a body but rather pure consciousness, became a source of considerable comfort for me. My body may die and decay, but my spirit would enter another realm, a higher state of being. What puzzles we are handed to solve on planet Earth. What challenges we have to face in order to be gifted with a sense of peace, and to finally experience a deeper understanding of who we really are.

I thought a lot about dying in the weeks that followed. I remembered my friend, Bobby, who had died of AIDS in 1990. During one of our long talks, I remember asking him whether he was afraid to die. He told me that he had no fear of death itself, because in the numerous recorded cases of clinical death, no one wanted to return to life on Earth. Everyone felt drawn to some indescribable place filled with pure love, light and sensations far beyond anything we can even begin to imagine. The only thing to fear, then, was the path one might travel in the process of reaching that other side. Bobby had a lot of trouble getting out of his body. He was ready to go long before he finally made the transition. That was something I could barely allow myself to ponder.

During the next few days my work gave me a sense of normalcy. If life went on as usual, I wagered, nothing could really be different. Everyone at work was unbelievably support-ive. I soon learned that three other women at my school were breast cancer survivors. At first the number seemed dispropor-tionate, until I remembered the "one-in-eight" formula and did the math.

Sunday rolled around, and the thought of attending church seemed almost magnetic. My whole family decided to go to services, which was very unusual. Stan had not been comfortable with organized religion for some time, and my stepdaughter, Margaret, usually attended her own church.

Did this gesture of attending church with me mean that everyone thought I was on my way out? I wondered. Whatever their reasons, I was glad they were there, glad we were together. The pew felt cozy, and my fears were the farthest thing from my mind during the service. When the time came for the congregation to share joys and concerns, one of my friends in the choir stood up and requested prayers for "someone" who would be facing surgery on Tuesday. By now almost everyone knew, but I was somehow happy not to actually hear my name. My personal prayers that day were directed at having cancer-free lymph nodes and for the strength to face whatever the future held. Even though my fears had taken a hike, I knew they were lying in wait just outside the church door.

Later that day, Stan and I went for a walk. Fall had replaced summer, and the maple leaves were breathtaking in their display of every shade of red and gold. I looked at the change of seasons differently than ever before. The brilliant, multicolored leaves were at the apex of their beauty, yet they were, in fact, dying. Soon they would fall to the earth and decay, and a breath of wind would scatter their remains. Without fear of impending death, they simply flowed with the rhythm of the universe, moving gently and naturally through the seasons. I hoped that if I did die, I could be beautiful, at least in spirit—bright and beautiful as the autumn leaves.

I had seen many deaths in the last two years while volunteering at *Our House of Portland*, a residential facility for people with AIDS. Despite its pain and heartbreak, *Our House* was vital and alive with love and compassion. Death, I discovered, has many faces. Some people were understandably angry, some became reclusive, and some remained outgoing and cheerful, even taking their meals at the dinner table until the last few days of their lives. One of the residents, Lee Joseph, will live forever in my heart. He had no hair, and his skull bore the scars from brain surgery. I'm sure he had his share of pain. AIDS has no mercy as it slowly and insidiously robs its victims of their lives. But through it all, Lee Joseph maintained a quiet dignity, a certain quality that virtually brought me to my knees in admiration. Knowing he was dying, he was keeping a journal of the last chapter of his life. When typing was too strenuous, he would speak into a tape recorder. One day I told him that I had heard death compared to taking off a tight pair of shoes. He immediately went to his room and entered what I had said into his journal. Lee remained interested in life and continued to read and study almost up until his death. He never seemed down, and it was always a pleasure to be in his company. If my death was looming on the horizon, I hoped I could take it in my stride and perhaps be an inspiration to someone, as Lee Joseph had been to me.

Monday was a typical work day. My supervisor had offered me the option of taking an extra day of sick leave, but too much time to reflect on my situation didn't seem prudent.

My students held my interest and occupied my time. No day in special education is ever boring. As we assisted our students one by one onto the little yellow buses, I found myself wishing the day didn't have to end. Maybe if I just stayed at school, this would all go away. But the shadows of night loomed ahead...countdown to God only knew what.

Hoping to avoid a fitful night, I gulped down an over-the-counter sleep aid and changed into a night shirt. Standing in front of the upstairs mirror, I suddenly felt a rush of sorrow. This would be the last night on earth for my breast. Finally, I felt the need for a long, hard look at myself. The bruises and the stitches from the biopsy stared back at me accusingly. They evoked a wave of sadness, even a distinct, and at the same time, nebulous, touch of guilt. My breast had been part of my body, part of who I was, and tomorrow the surgeon would slice it from my chest and send it off to the lab like a piece of meat from a butcher shop. I looked hard at my reflection in the mirror—I would never see myself like this again. Tears began to well up in my eyes, and the words formed almost inaudibly, "I'm so sorry...it wasn't supposed to be this way."

3

Flowers,
Friends,
and Aspirations

*"If you come at four o'clock, then at three o'clock,
I shall begin to be happy."*

—Antoine de Saint-Exupery
from *The Little Prince*

My daughter, Margaret, arrived early on the morning of the 15th. What a blessing she had been to me through all of this turmoil. Like a burst from a flower on an icy winter day, she had magically brightened my life. The day after I had called her with the dismal results of my biopsy, she had made arrangements to take time off from work and take care of Mama while I was in the hospital. Margaret had a natural way with elderly people. She knew exactly what to say, how to be comforting and reach Mama's fragile state of comprehension and reason. I was overwhelmed by my daughter's expression of love. With her loving presence in the house, I knew everything would be under control. I hadn't known how I would possibly manage caring for my mother while recuperating from major surgery. For one thing, she didn't really understand what was happening and would be needing constant guidance and reassurance.

I had finally told her that some of the cells of my breast tissue didn't look healthy, and my doctor recommended the mastectomy just to be safe. From that day on, every time I returned from work, she would ask, "Did you have your operation?"

Perhaps Mama would think my absence was due to my work for the next few days.

Time to go!

Margaret and I exchanged a big hug and clung to each other in silence for a moment. I broke away from her and followed Stan out into the early morning fog. The grayness of the morning air suited my mood. I felt just as colorless and shrouded in obscurity as this early winter day. I wondered what my future would hold. I wanted to stop my thoughts, stop that bleak, dismal mood, and I felt mildly relieved when we pulled up to the hospital entrance.

This was it! This was where it would happen.

After checking into the hospital we were ushered to a room by a kind, elderly volunteer. The countdown was on. I tried to keep the conversation light. Poor Stan was obviously shaken. No way now to get away, no way to deny what was about to happen.

A nurse arrived at my side and asked me several health-related questions. No allergies, no illnesses, no family history of cancer? No. Nothing. But I was changing that, wasn't I? I was adding a new chapter to our family history. Silence hovered after she left and closed the door behind her.

The air seemed unusually cold. Barbara had given me a cuddly, hot-pink oversize velour robe, and I decided to wear it over my chic, chilly, open-ended hospital gown. As I pulled the warm, soft fabric around my shivering frame, I could almost feel Barbara standing beside me. She'd be praying for me right about now, and knowing that meant everything in the world to me.

A few minutes passed, and Barbara's sister-in-law, Kathi, appeared at the door. I'd forgotten she worked at the hospital. Kathi had lost both parents and one brother to cancer. I was touched that she had come. She greeted me with genuine warmth and affection.

"What time is your surgery?" she asked. Tears were glistening her eyes.

"It's been moved to two o'clock, but I don't expect the surgery to be on time. They appear to be pretty backed up." I attempted to sound casual. We chatted comfortably for a while about and around everything and nothing. She didn't stay long, but I'll always remember that she took the time to see me. A familiar face was like a ray of sunshine, a welcome change amidst all the questions and needles.

Presently two young interns arrived on the scene and inquired whether I would object to answering a few questions. I quickly agreed to what seemed to be another welcome interruption of this endless, nervous waiting. The young doctors-to-be asked their questions with the well-acquired air of professional detachment.

"Any cancer in your family?"

"Only a paternal aunt. Ovarian cancer."

"Are you a smoker?"

"Not since 1975."

"Do you drink coffee?"

"Sometimes. Usually tea."

"How and when was your cancer discovered?"

"In late October. I had a routine mammogram."

"No palpable lump?"

"No."

"When was your biopsy?"

"A week ago."

"Anything occur between then and now?"

"No, other than finding out I'd be losing my breast."

"It's a small price to pay to save your life."

Until the young intern's last comment, the exchange had felt more like filling out a questionnaire. His words didn't set well with me. How about if we put his family jewels on the chopping block? Maybe then he could determine the relative importance of losing a body part. This guy definitely needed some sensitivity training, but I knew that if I responded, I'd lose control. Looking back, I wish I had simply told him how I felt. No woman who is facing a terrifying disfigurement wants her pain minimized by someone who has never walked in her shoes. Maybe I should have spoken up and saved some other woman from a similar experience. Good doctors should know these things. Oh well, not today.

Some time later the hospital minister showed up and asked whether I'd like for him to pray with me. When I said that I would, he asked if there was anything in particular I wanted mentioned. Clear lymph nodes, of course, were my chief concern. His soothing prayer was like a hug from God. His words went something like this:

God, we know you're everywhere, and you'll be there before the surgeon's knife does its work. We join in prayer today for healthy lymph nodes and for healing wherever it's needed.

For some reason, I always feel as though the prayers of other people, especially pastors and other "religious professionals," carry more clout with God than do my own. The last few days had found me calling everyone I knew in the world who could add my name to a prayer list anywhere.

Finally a nurse started an I.V. in my arm, and I was wheeled into pre-op. The dimly lit room was filled with people waiting to be sliced up one way or another. Strangely enough, it all seemed amusing. Maybe the tranquilizers were kicking in, or maybe it was just a case of nerves. My sense of misguided humor often breaks through under pressure. I remember having spent the greater portion of my dad's funeral squelching uncontrollable laughter. Of course, the Benevolent and Protective Order of Elks, God bless them, hadn't helped when they called his name and waited for a response from the coffin. I had thought about lowering my voice and answering, "Here," but I resisted the urge in deference to my grieving mother. I never cried until I saw my dad's hat hanging in the hall closet a few days later. Then I thought I would never stop.

My anesthesiologist was great. She explained what she would be doing, and we got into a conversation about the possible relationship between stress and breast cancer. We both laughed and agreed that our jobs left us wide open for unanticipated "breast reduction."

The next thing I knew, I was waking up in a private room banked with beautiful flowers. Stan had brought several pink and white lilies, and their delicate fragrance permeated the room. My pain was minimal, and the bandages were as thick as the breast on my left side had been. A nurse came in and explained the patient-controlled analgesic (P.C.A.) P.C.A. is a welcome innovation for all surgery patients. The painkiller is connected to a button which the patient can push at will, and the nurses love it because it saves them a lot of time. The fact that the patient never needs to call for a pain shot, offers a measure of control. The system only dispenses a certain amount of the medication every ten minutes, but it eliminates the anxiety of having to wait in pain until a nurse becomes available.

The aftereffects of surgery itself certainly weren't as severe as I had anticipated. I ate part of my dinner and decided to go for a walk. Getting up gingerly, I dragged my I.V. pole around the nurses' station several times and then returned to my room.

The phone rang. Ruthie, my friend from Bellingham, was on the line. She was surprised to hear me sound so chipper already. I figured I must be doing pretty well. After all, she had seen a few mastectomies in her many years of nursing.

"I can't believe you're up and around," she exclaimed with obvious delight.

"I feel great. This P.C.A. routine you told me about is a kick. I love it." We talked for several minutes and then hung up. I dozed off again into the euphoria of morphine.

The nurses were nothing short of saints. I had heard horror stories about overworked, crabby nurses, but these were happy and caring beings, and I loved them all. Even my busy anesthesiologist, Janice, stopped by to chat.

"How did I do?" she asked me, a quick smile in her eyes.

"You did great! I didn't wake up once," I responded with a grin.

How nice of her to stop by. Little things like Janice's visit can really do a lot to lighten the load. She didn't have to take the time to see me, but she did, and I'll always remember her for it. These are the little unsolicited acts of kindness that we hold in our hearts forever.

I spent the remainder of the evening talking to my friends on the telephone. What can I say? It was getting boring. Stan swears I'll wake up some day with a telephone growing out of my ear. It *would* be more convenient, I must say!

The following morning I was able to talk my doctor into sending me home. I certainly wouldn't advise such an early release for everyone, but for me it seemed right at the time. It made me feel more normal. The flip side of the coin was that the moment I walked in my door, I assumed the responsibility of caregiver. Elder care isn't always easy even when we're well, let alone when it's coupled with the stress of cancer surgery and its many psychological challenges.

As I sat in one of the overstuffed chairs in the living room, I was aware of an uncomfortable feeling in my chest. It wasn't really a pain, just discomfort, not unlike the feeling of having someone push hard against my incision with an open palm. Two drains hung from beneath my bandages collecting body fluids. They looked for all the world like two small hand grenades. I had been given verbal and written instructions explaining how to empty them and record the amounts of fluid which had accumulated. I could hardly wait.

The dogs were overjoyed to see me, and Chelsea, the larger dog, eventually bounded onto my lap and collided with my chest. Surprisingly, the pain was insignificant. The doctor had given me a prescription for pain medication, but so far I hadn't needed any.

Before long, some of the people from my church began to call and ask Stan about my condition. No one expected me to be home yet. Two or three people visited later that day, and flowers arrived from the choir, my school and several close friends. I love flowers, and our living room took on a cheerful air as I arranged and rearranged the bouquets. The mailbox was stuffed with get-well cards, some from people in Yreka who I wouldn't have thought remembered me. It was all very humbling.

As the afternoon shadows chased away the midday sun, I could feel myself winding down. The dull feeling of pressure in my chest changed to a sort of burning sensation, and I took a couple of pain pills. After dinner I helped Mama to change her clothes and saw her to her bed. Then I climbed the stairs to turn in for the day. The lilies Stan had given me looked beautiful on the dresser. I loved their fragrance and delighted in the thought that he had picked them out just for me.

My thoughts drifted to the past and to our twenty-six years together. The time spent in New York and the years after we had returned to Portland and decided to settle there were woven into a patchwork of memories. I remembered watching him on stage at the rehearsals of Portland Opera and the New Savoy (Gilbert and Sullivan) Company. His voice was a resonant "spinto" like none I had ever heard, and I was so proud that he was my husband. Sometimes I could hardly believe it was real, that I was actually married to this fine singer-actor, this man who, when he appeared in even a small buffo role, transfixed his audience as though he were the only performer on stage.

This was a good man, someone with depth of character. When my mother had begun to become forgetful and we realized she could no longer remain alone in her apartment, it was Stan who had been adamant that she should live with us. And it was Stan who took care of her while I was at work, setting her up with little jobs to keep her busy and taking her for rides in the country to raise her spirits.

I thought back to the time I had called him from work and asked him to pick up a dying cat. The poor animal had wandered into the parking lot so weak she could hardly walk.

I didn't want her to die alone. Stan arrived within a few minutes with a blanket and a box. When I came home, he was sitting next to her on our deck reading a book. I knew he had been there all afternoon keeping her company, making sure she had water and a soft place to rest.

And now he was standing by me as I faced my mortality. I knew he would be by my side when I needed him, despite my disfigurement. He probably wouldn't give me a great deal of verbiage, and I wouldn't always be privy to his feelings, but I knew the important piece. I knew, without a doubt, that he would be there.

The next morning I decided I was long overdue for a bath. Bathing without soaking the bandages was a feat for Harry Houdini. I tried putting the drains on the side of the bathtub. All went well for a few minutes until one fell off. Now there's a painful experience! When I finished scraping myself off the ceiling, I got out of the bathtub and dried myself. What a wretched little ritual to anticipate day after day. Stan finally came up with the ingenious idea of putting a belt around my neck and attaching the drains to the buckle. It worked perfectly.

Eventually my bandages needed to be changed. Looking at one's chest is part of the healing process, so I'd been told. Having seen Aunt Ruby's scars several times, I felt ready for the unveiling. Let me go on record as saying that nothing could have prepared me for what I was about to see. My incision had been stapled! My chest was grinning obscenely at me, like a big mouth with braces. This then, was the price I paid for my decision not to request the services of a plastic surgeon to close the wound.

Reapplying the bandages proved nearly impossible due to the lack of mobility in my left arm. Reluctantly I summoned Stan. He may as well see it. We were both stuck with it for the time being. I watched his face, but his expression gave me no clue as to what he felt. At least he didn't ask for a barf bag. That was something. Then a strange thing happened. My knees started to buckle, and my head started to swim. The only thing I could do was drop to the floor. In a few minutes the sensation passed. Was it something physical, or was it emotional shock? Ah, the mystery of the mastectomy. Such an enchanting experience!

Part of it *was* enchanting. Birthday cards and get-well cards filled our mailbox daily, and the phone rang nonstop. I was basking in the sunshine of love and attention. Barbara, knowing my fondness for animals, sent me a wonderful bouquet complete with little "endangered species" Christmas tree ornaments — a little gorilla was sucking his thumb. My new friends now occupy the ledge of the kitchen window the year round. Penny called nearly every day and even offered to spend time with Mama.

I still remember Penny's get-well card. She wrote that if it would ease my pain, she'd spend $1,000 a month on phone calls or walk in raw sewage up to her knees. My kind of friend! One of my other cards was from Alyce, another educational assistant at my school. She said that two years ago she had received the same frightening news and that if she could be of any help, she'd be glad to talk with me. Alyce eventually proved to be a Godsend.

Waiting to hear the results of my lymph nodes dissection was the longest forty-eight hours I've spent in my life. Ask any woman who has been through it. If the nodes are clear, the prognosis is about 25 percent better. That's a huge difference. People with positive nodes can often be cured, but it is a lot more serious because the cancer has obviously spread. Positive nodes usually mean having to undergo chemotherapy.

The anxiously awaited call came the day before my birthday, and it was undeniably the best birthday gift of my life. My lymph nodes were cancer-free. The nurse told me that these were the phone calls she loved to make. My feet didn't touch the floor as I flew up the stairs to tell Stan. He was more than relieved.

After the pathology report was in, it was time to discuss treatment or adjuvant therapy, as it is called. I had read about the various kinds of chemo and radiation therapies and knew that I might not lose my hair even if chemotherapy proved necessary. Still, the thought of sending poisons into my system to kill some of my cells was very sobering to me, because healthy cells are destroyed in the process as well, and the immune system is compromised. By far the most frightening aspect was the thought that the treatments might be unnecessary. Doctors can run tests that provide certain indices as to the probability of the spread of cancer, but they can never be sure that even when all the tests come back negative, the patient is completely cured. Because we don't yet have truly definitive tests, a perfectly healthy person could be receiving chemo or radiation treatments just to be on the safe side. For that reason I was greatly relieved when my doctor prescribed hormone therapy instead. Apparently this is the best thing available for node-negative women who are post-menopausal with fairly non-aggressive tumors caught in the early stages.

Just the same, I decided to obtain additional opinions. Whatever treatment was chosen, would be, as I understood it, my one chance for a cure. To err could mean death. In addition to asking my G.P., I arranged for a consultation with an oncologist. All three doctors concurred. The hormone most frequently prescribed for breast cancer treatment is Tamoxifen, which blocks estrogen to the breast and binds to the estrogen receptors on breast cancer cells to prevent growth, i.e., gene transcription. Much like estrogen, Tamoxifen is also thought to protect the bones and heart. The most serious side effect is an increased chance of endometrial cancer, and the most uncomfortable side effect is hot flashes. The drug costs about $100 a month. Thank God for health insurance.

~~~~~~~~~~~

Trips to the doctor's office during the ensuing weeks were all too frequent. In an attempt to prove to myself that nothing had changed, I started jogging ten days after surgery. As a result, fluid continued to accumulate on my chest wall long after the drains had been removed. This necessitated aspirating the buildup of fluids with a long needle that reminded me of a poultry baster. The first time my doctor brandished the needle, I nearly wet my pants, but the procedure proved to be quite painless after all. My chest area and the inside of my arm were almost totally numb.

My doctor practiced at three different locations, two of which were quite a distance from our home. The long ride back and forth to his office began to wear on me even more than the twice-weekly aspirations. Every three or four days, Stan and I fought the traffic to keep another date with the giant needle. I felt trapped keeping pace with this endless treadmill. Why was I complaining? Chemotherapy and radiation must be a thousand times worse.

My doctor told me that the incision would need to be sufficiently healed before he would write a prescription for a prosthesis, so I decided to embark on a "falsie" expedition. The *Yellow Pages* provided me with several choices, one of which was a small bra boutique on our side of town. I got into the car and wondered, "What next?" The small shop turned out to be a friendly place with a saleswoman who dealt with women like me every day and had a reassuring manner about her. She sold me some bra pads and then showed me a prosthesis or two that might serve my future needs. It's amazing what has been created to cover up the loss of a woman's breast. She introduced me to a variety of prostheses, one especially clever because it can be attached directly to the body with velcro. What ever did we do before velcro?

The velcro idea was of interest to me because I rarely wore a bra, and the idea of having to strap on my boobs didn't appeal to me in the least. The prosthesis she showed me felt exactly like real flesh. Several types of mastectomy bras were available, most containing pockets for pads or prostheses. I bought a bra but couldn't wear it for long because the drain scar was directly under the bra line and caused considerable discomfort. Another thing to keep in mind in any kind of breast surgery is to ask—no, insist—that the drain exit be placed below the bra line. I later found out that it could easily be done — no problem!

Velcro is wonderful but very expensive. One strip to anchor a prosthesis costs five dollars and lasts only three or four days. Velcro is not practical for women suffering from hot flashes. The chest area simply doesn't remain dry enough to keep the adhesive securely in place, as I later discovered, much to my embarrassment.

My hot flashes were relentless, and besides being uncomfortable, they proved to be an hourly reminder that I'd had breast cancer. Poor Stan. I changed from someone who was always cranking up the heat to an overheated basket case. All through the night I threw off the covers as I tossed and turned and wiped the rivers of sweat from my chest and forehead. I found myself rushing out onto our deck nude in the middle of winter. Fortunately we had built a six-foot fence for privacy. The sight of a lopsided naked woman would probably have been too much for some of our neighbors.

After several weeks my incision had healed well, and my chest wall was no longer retaining fluid, so I made an appointment with the mastectomy consultant at a local department store in order to be fitted for a prosthesis. Pinning falsies to my undershirt was beginning to get on my nerves, and I desperately wanted something more realistic. Up until this time, wearing form-fitting sweaters and clinging shirts had been out of the question. I hoped a prosthesis would allow me to expand my wardrobe.

I arrived promptly for my appointment with the consultant, who proved to have the perfect personality for her job. She put me at ease immediately. I left the store wearing velcro and a new prosthesis and carrying a bag of fancy, expensive undershirts. What a grand feeling! No more baggy two-pocketed plaids from the men's department.

Six weeks after surgery I returned to work. Ten weeks

after surgery I was luxuriating in the delicious foam of a fragrant bubble bath when I felt a small lump in my right breast. This just couldn't be happening—but it was.

I froze. My mind shut down. I was isolated in a vacuum of nothingness. Except for a fast-rising tidal wave of pure panic radiating one thousand degrees, I felt paralyzed.

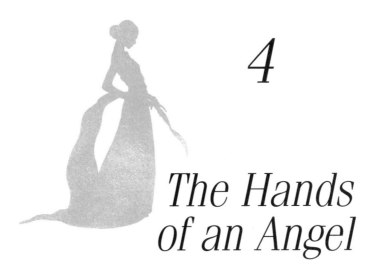

4

The Hands
of an Angel

*"An angel will appear in whatever
manner you see it."*

—Emmanuel's Book III

My doctor was certain that the new lump was only a swollen duct and told me not to touch it and to come back in two weeks. How could he be so confident? Two weeks later nothing had changed, and I found myself back in mammography, clamped in the familiar iron jaws of the X-ray machine. Standing there naked to the waist and totally powerless suddenly evoked my fury. Then a rather astonishing thought flashed through my head. What good was one breast anyway? I was already disfigured. It would be nice to be able to wander around the house in a nightshirt or T-shirt without feeling the need to put on a prosthesis to even out my chest.

The idea of being symmetrical again seemed extremely appealing. For the remainder of my life the yearly nightmare of having a mammogram and worrying about the results could be eliminated. No breasts, no mammograms. At that moment I seriously considered the possibility of having my right breast removed. What a relief to realize that I could jump through one less medical hoop. The choice was mine.

The following week at school, I made my final decision. Up to that point I had been anchoring my prosthesis to my chest with a V-shaped strip of velcro purchased at the Nordstrom mastectomy department. I liked the appearance and appreciated being braless again, even though my toasty hot-flash episodes had made the area moist with perspiration. I was aware of the impending difficulty of keeping the velcro strips securely attached to a moist surface, but the desire to avoid pocketing my "breast" in an uncomfortable mastectomy bra had kept me in partial denial, and I continued to forge ahead with the convenience and aesthetic advantage of velcro. Then came the *moment of truth.*

We were sitting in the school library: my friend, Becky, myself, and a group of students from our classroom. Suddenly, something didn't feel right. My prosthesis had come loose and was sliding down my chest. Thank God my blouse was tucked in, or it would have probably gone bouncing across the floor in full view of twenty high school students. After discreetly pushing the wandering silicone breast back into place and anchoring it with my forearm, I leaned over to Becky and whispered into her ear, "Beck, can you watch the kids for a minute? My boob just fell off."

We both started laughing. The more we tried to keep quiet, the more we laughed. Soon we were gasping for air, and tears were running down our cheeks. Our kids, sensing the humor of it all, started to laugh at the top of their lungs. The librarian was visibly disgusted, and every set of eyes in the room was focused directly on our undignified, noisy table. Wishing I could make myself invisible, I slunk out the door and headed for the restroom. Fortunately I had an extra bra in my locker for just such an emergency. From then on out, I decided that wearing the velcro-attached prosthesis was too risky. One of the draw-backs of having another mastectomy was the idea of then need-ing two five-dollar velcro strips every four days instead of one. Seventy-five dollars a month was pretty steep for my budget. The removal of my right breast seemed more and more logical.

As long as a bra was necessary, why not "strap it ALL on" and be safe and symmetrical? Breast tissue hadn't done me any favors. Why not just be done with it?

At some point during this anxious, worrisome time, one of my doctors ordered a needle biopsy on my right breast—the same procedure that my regular physician had recommended in 1991. This seemed prudent, in view of the fact that we had wasted more than three years, three precious years, when my surgeon had decided against it in 1991.

The needle biopsy involved the use of a screen, something similar to an ultrasound transducer, and a needle. When the technician popped the needle in, he apparently ruptured a cyst, because it disappeared from the screen completely. That may be nothing out of the ordinary, but it rattled my nerves. What if he had just released malignant cells to invade other areas of my body? Ignorance is not always bliss.

When he was finished, I could still feel the lump in my breast, so he must have exploded something else. An excisional biopsy was, to me, the only logical answer. If it proved to be anything serious, an immediate mastectomy would be in order. Otherwise surgery would be scheduled in the summer when being absent from school was not an issue.

Because my surgeon was unavailable, another doctor was scheduled to do my next examination. She was a delightful young woman with an absolutely magnetic personality. She listened intently as I explained that even though I had made a definite decision to have another mastectomy in the summer, I wanted a biopsy now to set my mind at ease. When I had finished talking, she was quiet for a moment and then said, "If you're really planning to have a mastectomy, why not do it now and be done with it? The recovery for a simple mastectomy is only five days."

Apparently as long as the lymph nodes aren't involved, the recovery is much easier than with a modified radical operation. The arm doesn't become stiff and sore, and only one drain is necessary. I didn't need time to reflect.

"Let's schedule it," I blurted out quickly before I could change my mind.

The wheels were set in motion, and surgery was scheduled for the following week.

The drive home was euphoric. No more fear of cancer in the right breast. Worrying about a recurrence of any kind was bad enough. Breast cancer can spread to the liver, lungs, brain and bones, not in any particular order. Every cough, every upset stomach, every possible symptom sent me into a temporary panic attack. This would be one less thing to fear.

After hearing my mounting frustration and terror, Stan began to see my side of the story, and at least partially, was coming to understand my decision. A few weeks after my first surgery we had watched a documentary featuring a woman who had decided to have a double mastectomy even though only one breast was cancerous. We had both remarked that we didn't understand her reasoning. Why would she remove a healthy breast? Now I understood her action completely. Even though Stan still struck me as being somewhere in the middle, he supported my decision.

Some of my friends wondered if I was being a bit hasty and worried openly about future regrets and the possibility of aftershock. I remember having dinner with Darlene, one of the teachers with whom I had worked a few years back. She remarked that I seemed to be treating the whole experience as though I'd just had a tooth extracted.

What she didn't suspect was the fact that most of my bravado was feigned, born out of my desire to appear outwardly strong. Even my closest friends often mistook it for real courage or even indifference. Darlene said that I should think long and hard before undergoing the ordeal of another mastectomy. Her concern was understandable. I would have entertained the same thoughts had the situation been reversed.

But I really was comfortable with my decision and never looked back. On March 10, 1995, I said good-bye to my right breast. This experience was entirely different. For one thing, the lump was relatively sure to be benign. For another, I had already tested the waters. This wasn't a mystery. I knew that the pain after surgery was mild and easily managed.

When I came out of the recovery room, Stan returned home to tend to Mama, and Penny arrived and spent most of the evening with me. We were joined for a while by Kelli, one of my friends from *Our House of Portland.* Kelli is a licensed massage therapist who volunteers at the hospice one or more nights a week, providing therapeutic massage to people in the final stages of AIDS. She massaged my legs and feet as we visited. Between Kelli's hands and the P.C.A., I'd never felt better. Finally my friends left and I drifted off into la-la land.

As the morning sun peeked through the window, my doctor stopped by and gave the okay for my release. An hour later Stan and Margaret came and drove me home. The entire twenty-four hours had been comfortable. Nothing sad, no regrets, just relief.

This surgery required only one drain, but even so, my chest wall filled with fluid and required several aspirations. Knowing what to expect proved helpful. Also, I was able to schedule most of my appointments at Good Samaritan Hospital, a short drive I could comfortably make alone.

A few days after the surgery the bandages were ready to come off. I braced myself, knowing that if any part of this would be difficult, it would be looking at my incision. Carefully dislodging the tape, I peeked tentatively at my new chest. Then a smile broke across my face. My doctor had taken the time to use subcutaneous sutures and had secured the incision with tiny pieces of tape. The difference was phenomenal. Instead of feeling hideous, I felt cared for, as though an angel had descended from Heaven and closed my wound with her divine breath. In my mind, my doctor really was an angel, and I'll never forget her for as long as I live. The scar healed in a barely noticeable, straight line—a sharp contrast to the "teeth marks" on my left side.

A week after surgery I returned to work. In retrospect it was too soon, given the physical demands of my job. Some students in our classroom had to be lifted out of wheelchairs and positioned for physical therapy. My co-workers offered to do my lifting, but I often refused help, not wanting to appear weak. All went reasonably well until the day we were transporting students downstairs on the freight elevator. As I closed the door, I jerked the big leather door straps with unrestrained vigor. Pain shot through my chest, and for a minute I froze, almost afraid to move. The pain subsided, but that evening I felt the fluid rising and accumulating in my chest wall. The skin had been separated where it had healed to the chest. This would no doubt mean a whole new round of rendezvous with the giant needle. Would this medical merry-go-round ever stop?

~~~~~~~~~~~

That year, spring break fell somewhere in March, and Stan and I decided to get away to the beach. Margaret agreed to stay with Mama, so we loaded the dogs into the car and hit the coast highway. Time alone at last...just us, the dogs and the ocean. As we rounded the big curve between Cannon Beach and Manzanita, the endless ocean glistened under a blue sky and stretched in all its majesty to the far-away horizon. I could hardly wait to get out of the car and smell the air. We arrived at our oceanfront motel and unloaded the car. Suddenly we were in Shangri-La, a carefree wonderland away from the pressure of life's trials and daily demands.

I have yet to go anywhere without forgetting something important—this time it was my Tamoxifen. If that were to happen to me today, I wouldn't give it a second thought. But for the first year or so after my surgeries, I was afraid to miss even one pill. We had to find a pharmacy and beg for a few days' supply of my medication. We ended up in the tiny town of Wheeler. While we were waiting for the pharmacist to fill my request, we browsed through books and magazines, and a small book on menopause caught my eye.

I decided to buy it for something to read. Big mistake! One of the chapters contained some information on breast cancer. The words jumped off the page: "Breast cancer strikes one in eight women in America, and its seriousness can in no way be overstated." It went on to say that most women afflicted with the disease eventually die from it. I started to cry. Up to this point I believed that my prognosis was good and that I would probably live to a ripe old age. This bit of information hit me harder than the actual diagnosis. What I didn't think to consider was the fact that my problem had been discovered very early, which may not be the case for the vast majority of breast cancer patients.

In retrospect I realize how much I was caught up in myself. "My" cancer, "My" misfortune, "My" uncertain future, etcetera, etcetera, etcetera. Instead of controlling my thinking, I was allowing IT to control ME.

When we returned to our motel I went into the bathroom and locked the door. Crouching on the cold floor next to the toilet, I attempted to muffle my sobs. Our get-away holiday was as good as ruined for me, but I wanted Stan to enjoy himself. The last few months had been hard on him as well, and he needed this change of scenery. I dried my tears and washed my face with cold water. "At least I'm alive today," I thought.

The sunset in progress was breathtaking, but it might as well have been a dark thunder cloud I was watching. I plopped myself on the bed and reached for the trusty remote. Good old TV, the American sedative, the people's pacifier.

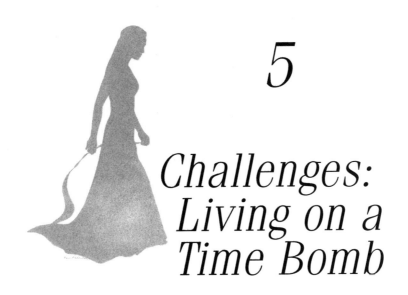

5

Challenges:
Living on a
Time Bomb

"Happiness is a choice, not a response."

— Kathleen Russell and Larry Wall
from *Achieve Your Dreams*

At some point my dream ended, and the stark reality of living day-to-day on a potential time bomb took hold of me.

Living without estrogen made me edgy and unfocused, and the fears associated with having had breast cancer added fuel to the fire of the menopausal furnace. Relentless hot flashes drove me to the point of madness. More and more frequently, I had to dash out of the house, heading straight for the deck and the soothing comfort of the cool, fresh air. My steamy, sweaty body could have melted an iceberg.

During the first two years after surgery the thought of cancer was never far from my mind. Any attempt to redirect my thoughts proved futile. The minute I opened my eyes in the morning, fear and anxiety came rushing in, seizing my very soul as the battle to go on with my life continued to push me to the limits. Because I've always believed that our words and thoughts attract our circumstances, my constant fear was that this endless mind trip of mine might be opening the door to a recurrence. Catch 22— alive and in full color.

Hoping to increase my odds of staying alive, I was compulsively investing in vitamins and herbs by the carload. Our regular food supply was being crowded out of our cupboards and off the shelves with my acquisition of "health" stuff. A kombucha tea preparation took up residence in the refrigerator. Stan was disgusted. He remarked on more than one occasion that every time he opened the fridge, he expected to be attacked by the slimy, unattractive yeast formation floating at the surface of its glass container. I admit that it was pretty scary looking, but it tasted great and provided me with some measure of mental security.

Frantically, I added anything rumored to be anti-carcinogenic to my growing intake of daily "requirements," hoping to keep cancer on the run. *(This is by no means meant to infer that supplemental natural remedies are not effective in preventing recurrence. I really believe in their value and continue to use a number of them as directed by my naturopath.)*

Reading about cancer had become another of my obsessions. Before long every book dealing with the subject of the disease and its cures was making its way onto the shelves of our library. Some books helped, but some only served to compound my fears. (See recommended reading list on page 99.)

Soon, however, I began to discover more pleasant ways to further my overall healing process. Resting in a comfortable position in a darkened room listening to guided meditations seemed to have a positive effect on my psyche. Bookstores are filled with these tapes, and you can design an individual program to fit your needs. Some of my favorite tapes were by the Simonton Cancer Center and by Louise Hay. I struggled to learn to meditate on my own (without guidance from others), but I had trouble focusing and was unable to take more than two breaths without letting my bout with cancer creep defiantly to the surface. It is a known fact that people who meditate stay healthier and live longer, but I simply couldn't clear my mind.

I also noticed that other strange behaviors were beginning to invade my life. Daily tasks had become extremely difficult—an attention deficit made its presence known. One day I wrote down a telephone message and discovered later that something had caused me to stop in mid-sentence. Could it be dementia? Was it hereditary? Or had the cancer metastasized, starting its macabre dance in my brain? I was beginning to feel disabled, inferior. On a scale of one to ten, my faith, my positive attitude and my self-esteem didn't even register.

During this less-than-centered period in my life, I was blessed with having two guiding lights. Alyce and Laura, two friends from school, were both cancer survivors and had jumped through all of the fiery hoops of fear. They were both close at hand and always willing to help me through the hard times with words of encouragement and helpful information.

Laura had survived cancer for several years. I had seen her go through chemotherapy and radiation and had often wondered how she could "hang in there" so well. As we started talking more and more, she told me that she had been node-positive and that cancer had been found in three of her lymph nodes at the time of her surgery. Yet she seemed to be doing fine. Laura did a lot to validate my feelings. Life, she said, would never be the same, but it would eventually get better. A day never passed that she didn't think about cancer.

Alyce was my other mentor. She understood my fears and my inability to focus. Having watched her mother succumb to the disease, she was deathly afraid of a recurrence herself, but her life was improving day by day. Alyce was always there for me when I needed to talk. She and Laura acted as an on-site support group, always close by and always willing to help.

Communicating with my family wasn't always easy because the episode had been frightening for them as well, and they were eager to put it behind them. Stan once told me he thought I could get on with my life a lot faster if I'd stop talking about cancer so much. He may have been right, but doing that was like trying to stop scratching an annoying mosquito bite.

I just couldn't do it.

Alyce and Laura had been so supportive that I hoped I could at least do the same for other women in the future. My friends had given me strength and I felt strongly about passing it on. My chance came all too soon.

Some time around April, Darlene called me and said that she had been scheduled for a biopsy. She just wanted to know what to expect, and I told her what I knew from my experience. For some reason, the idea of a malignancy barely crossed my mind. If it had happened to me, then it wouldn't happen to her. The biopsy was just a safety measure to set her mind at ease.

A few days later Darlene's closest friend, Jan, telephoned to tell me the biopsy had come back positive. She informed me that Darlene didn't feel like talking right now but that she would call me soon. Darlene had cancer. The words froze in my mind. How could this be happening? They had to be wrong. Maybe someone messed up the pathology reports. If this were true, it meant we had been working side by side in 1991, both having breast cancer and both not knowing it. Was it something in the building or something about special ed? All I could really do in the beginning was keep her in my thoughts and prayers and let her know I'd be there if she ever felt the need to talk.

Darlene called me the following week. She'd been waking up in the middle of the night screaming. Her tumor was the size of an ice cube, and the doctor had told her she'd definitely have chemotherapy. A decision hadn't been made yet as to whether she would require a mastectomy.

On the day of Darlene's surgery, I decided to take some flowers to the hospital. She probably wouldn't want company, but I could leave them at the nurses' station. Jan happened to be there, and we had an opportunity to talk. She told me that Darlene had opted for a lumpectomy. I was glad she hadn't lost her breast. Cancer is bad enough without being disfigured. The idea of a mastectomy had been very disturbing to her.

Darlene came through surgery with flying colors and started chemotherapy. We talked to each other often, and one night we met for dinner at a Chinese restaurant. She had lost most of her hair and was sporting a baseball cap in lieu of a wig. For some reason we found a lot to laugh about. She told me about the day she had accidentally taken the hospital elevator down to the morgue. Realizing her mistake, she turned to another woman in the elevator and commented glibly, "We're not dead yet, but we're workin' on it!" The other woman apparently had failed to grasp the humor and looked at Darlene with utter disdain. I, on the other hand, found the whole story hilarious.

We chatted on about this, that and our "situation," of course, and toward the end of the meal, Darlene asked me whether I had plans to participate in the *Race for the Cure.* I had never heard of the event. Having been released from the hospital so soon after surgery, I had missed out on a few things. The *Reach for Recovery* people usually drop by to help women through the traumatic experience of breast surgery, and they provide patients with a wealth of useful information related to healing and regaining mental balance. But I had been anxious to get home to my mother.

From Darlene, I learned that the *Race for the Cure* is sponsored by the Susan G. Komen Breast Cancer Foundation, a group founded by the sister of Susan Komen, a young, vibrant woman who had lost her life to the disease. The foundation also sponsors the Survivor's Brunch, an event featuring several speakers and a fashion show, and *Komen Issues*, an intense workshop held in many major cities for survivors and other interested parties. The *Race for the Cure* in Portland is one of the biggest in the nation and raises thousands of dollars each year for the "cure." The throng of participating survivors sporting hot-pink hats, and the sight of all those women, each with her own story, is awe-inspiring.

My friend and I made plans to attend both the race and the brunch. I was so sad that Darlene had breast cancer, but I now felt a deep bond with her beyond the context of a mere friendship. Our backgrounds may not have been alike, and we may have viewed the experience in a different light, but now we both understood feelings that other women can only imagine. When it's all said and done, and we look back on our lives and those of others, we come to realize that everyone has carried a bundle—no exceptions. No one leaves the planet untouched by pain, disappointments and hard knocks. We all bear a few scars from bumping into life's unexpected turns. Our unexpected turn was breast cancer, and it brought us together...it is, I later discovered, a unique little club—the survivors club. We had just received our initiation.

As we walked to our cars, Darlene handed me a designer shopping bag containing a tape about healing and a T-shirt. I was touched by her gift, which she said was "just because." Coincidentally, the shirt was exactly like one I had ruined and had been missing almost to the point of mourning. It was gray and had a big pink heart across the front, and the words: "Teach Only Love, For That Is What You Are." The garment had been designed by my friend, Rob, for the *A Course in Miracles Center* in Portland. I could feel myself choking up. Acts of caring and expressions of love touched my heart now more than ever. We said our good-byes, and I watched as she disappeared into the evening mist. I said a silent prayer, "God, please let her be okay. Please help us to heal ourselves."

Driving home I thought about the mind-body connection. The words from the Bible, "As a man thinketh, so is he," had come to mind many times since my cancer journey had begun. After watching my dance teacher, Daryle, die of lymphosarcoma and having lost Aunt Ruby after a nineteen-year struggle with the disease, my thoughts were often deluged with fears relating to the "Big C."

Had my imagination caused my fears to materialize? Had my preoccupation with cancer brought on its manifestation? Maybe the new meditation tape would help. What a waste of energy. What a pity to spend so much time worrying. When I wasn't worrying about a recurrence, I was worrying about how much I worried. The only thing I didn't worry about much, for some reason, was my liver. Oh, I "protected" it with milk-thistle enzyme because I read somewhere that it was good for the liver, but I seldom imagined any metastasis to that area. Maybe it was because I didn't really know where the liver was located in order to be on guard for possible symptoms. How Stan stuck with me through all my anxiety and moodiness, I'll never know. He must have felt as though he was suddenly married to a total stranger. I'm so grateful to him. This was indeed the true test of his love.

Every three months I went for an examination. This pattern goes on for the first two years after surgery. When checkup time rolled around I worked myself into a virtual state of insanity. Chest X-rays, blood tests, chest exams for local recurrence—I dreaded every procedure. Each time I entered the Comprehensive Cancer Center, I felt as though I was walking under a threatening, black cloud.

Sometimes I wondered if it would all have gone away if the lump had never been detected. Foolish thoughts for modern medicine, no doubt. My doctor prescribed an antidepressant, but the only effect was that I had less energy and experienced more confusion.

With the advent of summer came ten weeks of freedom from my classroom routine. As much as I loved "my kids" and welcomed the unique demands of my job, I needed a break. For those ten weeks there would be no more lifting and no more feeling inadequate at work.

Still feeling slightly sorry for myself, I invested in a "happy present," a nearly new car. We'd been chugging along in Mother's 1977 Cutlass Supreme, but lately the repair bills had mounted until our old car owed us more than it was worth. We had to have reliable transportation, and I needed something livelier on the horizon than the possibility of my impending demise. After searching here and there, we bought a 1994 candy-apple-red Mercury Sable. It was beautiful, comfortable and above all, it was dependable.

Blessed at last with a set of good wheels, I planned a trip

to Yreka. My friend, Doris, was having a fiftieth birthday party, and I decided to surprise her and show up. Stan offered to take care of Mama during my absence. She could still manage relatively well with someone at her side to provide guidance and simple directions. Our new automobile came equipped with a tape deck, so I brought along some Chopin, and a few of my "healing" tapes and hit the road.

The trip was extremely relaxing. Yreka will always be home to me, though more than half my life has been spent in other, more populated places. It's a peaceful little town of about 6,000, nestled in the hills of northern California. We moved there in 1948 because my father had wanted to get out of Los Angeles with its foul smog and congested roads. He had often remarked that the city was no place to raise kids, and the longer I live the more I agree with him. My entire childhood was spent swimming in clear lakes and sparkling rivers and hiking in the hills which hug the safe, friendly little California town.

Hooper and June Maplesden, an inspiring couple I'd met at *Our House of Portland,* lived in Yreka and had invited me to stay with them. These good people had lost their son to AIDS at *Our House,* and had experienced more than their share of grief and sorrow. Being from the same town and sharing so much history had made us fast friends.

As soon as Yreka came into sight, powerful emotions rushed up from the depth of my soul. The gentle hills of this familiar little town reached out with strong, loving arms waiting to hold me and rock my battle-scarred body until my pain disappeared. My God, how I'd missed it all!

Before settling in at Hooper and June's, there were a few places I'd been longing to see. Like a homing pigeon I headed for our little white house on 601 Siskiyou Street. Even with the "For Sale" sign on the lawn, it felt that at any moment Mama would come through the door humming a familiar old hymn, or Dad would walk around the corner from the back yard with a cigarette in his hand and his car keys jingling in his pocket.

Mama hadn't hummed for the last two years, and I

missed it. Everything was so different now. Dad was gone, and Mom was someone I'd once known and somehow lost along the way. She looked the same, and her sweet, loving spirit was constant, but her mind and personality were somewhere else. Sometimes I found myself sitting alone and saying, "Mama, where did you go? How did this happen?" She had been my best friend, always right there, and now she was gone. But the little white house was still there, waiting for new owners to write their story of life within its walls.

My next rendezvous with the past was the Evergreen Cemetery. Dad was buried there, waiting among the oaks and evergreens for the day when my mother would once again be by his side. The old burial place was filled with pine cones and wild sweet peas, and due to the dry climate, very few of the plots were covered with grass. The feeling was earthy and natural, like the hills that rose gently toward the blue sky. Deer wandered in at dusk and at the break of day to nibble away on the fresh flowers that graced the newly opened graves. Dad loved nature and had once told me he would be more than happy to share his flowers with the deer when his time came.

I got my bearings and drove alongside his grave. Sunshine, like liquid gold, touched my father's headstone as I read the inscription, "Beloved Gene." The plot looked well kept. I had covered it with loads of barkdust on my last visit, and the weeds hadn't managed to take root. Crouching down in the summer heat, I began my usual one-way conversation with Dad.

"I miss you, Dad. Everything seems so hard lately, but I guess you already know that. Mother hardly recognizes me anymore, and last year I found out I had cancer, and now I'm really scared. Please ask God to help Mom. Her life is so hard now. Please ask Him to do something." I was the child again, asking my dad to make it all well. "Please?"

I sat alone on the cement ledge by his grave, letting my tears flow freely, making no attempt to curb my emotions. After a few minutes I felt better. There's nothing like a good cry. I inhaled deeply of the fragrant, clear mountain air, stretched and walked on.

Walking felt good. The reddish-brown dirt under my feet and the scent of juniper around me lent an aura of peace and nostalgia to the moment. A small mausoleum marked "Cawley" led me to my old friend, Bobby's grave. He had been buried next to his father, and his grave still had no marker. In the trunk of my car was a small cross which I intended to have Hooper help me set above the temporary metal marker. I stood for a while, nearly void of thought, drinking in the present moment. A warm breeze had come up, and a blue jay scolded in the distance. Bobby's laughter echoed on the breeze as I finally walked to the car. AIDS could never really take him from me. His spirit was too strong. Death doesn't diminish the people we love as long as we carry them in our hearts and keep their memories alive. I could almost feel Bobby beside me as I drove through the iron gates and down Evergreen Lane.

Hooper and June lived only a few blocks from the cemetery, but I detoured a bit to visit some other places from the past. Driving past the Jackson Street School triggered another flood of memories. Several years ago Bobby and I had met in Yreka for our twentieth class reunion. We had decided to take a late-night walk down memory lane and had eventually found ourselves sitting on the swings in the old schoolyard talking up a storm. If I'd had a brother, I'd have wanted him to be like Bobby. His sister was a lucky woman.

Pausing at the street corner we had crossed so many times, I wondered if his spirit was still close by. Somehow I thought so. One of the speakers at his memorial service had mentioned Bobby's wish, that after he died, he would be like Jiminy Cricket, sitting on people's shoulders "giving them the answers to life's questions." Maybe he'd be around to give me some answers some day. Lately, I'd felt long on questions and short on answers.

The Maplesden's place was almost directly across the street from the old schoolyard. The wooden house was surrounded by lush vegetation. Hooper and June had been watching for me and were waiting at the door with greetings and loving hugs. I instantly fell in love with their home. The spacious living area was built around a fireplace, and the garden could be seen through the large windows on the back wall. A picture of their son, John, was a focal point of the room. I remembered him in his room at *Our House*, his beautiful face made pale and gaunt by a ruthless, insidious disease which would eventually rob him of his life. And I remembered Hooper and June in their unending devotion to him as he lay dying. Parents just didn't come any better. They were as good as mine, and that was as good as it gets.

Hooper showed me to my room. For the first time in over a year, I felt totally relaxed. Sitting on the side of the bed, I took a moment to enjoy the solitude that greeted me. I would come back to it, but right now I wanted to walk into the flavor of Yreka. This was my town. These were my people.

First, we went on a tour of Hooper's garden. I kicked off my shoes and followed him to the back yard. He dug a carrot from the rich, dark soil, washed off bits of earth, and handed it to me with a grin. Cool, crunchy and sweet—even the carrots tasted better in Yreka.

Hooper, in his jeans and plaid shirt, reminded me somewhat of my dad. He had that same air of honesty and warm simplicity about him. No pretension. Just a gentle hard-working man, someone you'd instinctively trust with your life.

June was waiting inside with a big pitcher of fresh lemonade. She was a tall, strong woman with beautiful white hair and an irresistible twinkle in her eye. Losing her son to AIDS had made her a veritable crusader. She had made the best of a heart-wrenching situation. They both had. Their lives for the last three years had been rough, but they never complained. Instead they harnessed their energies to teach compassion and understanding in the memory of a son who was, and always would be, vitally alive in their hearts.

Dinner was meatless. I could have bet on it. I had told June to cook what they usually ate, and I would eat the vegetables, fruits and other non-meat items, but in deference to my animal-rights issues, she had avoided serving meat. Most of the vegetables were from their garden, and everything was delicious. We talked long into the evening. June would be going to Doris' fiftieth birthday party at the grange hall, while Hooper was working a booth at the county fair. I could hardly wait to revisit the fairgrounds. Finally my eyelids were losing their battle with gravity, so I excused myself and went to my room. Lying in the dark, reflecting on the events of the day, I suddenly realized what had been missing. Hot flashes had been missing! I couldn't recall a single one. The soft breeze and the chirping of the crickets singing under my window were the last sounds I held in my ears as I slipped blissfully into sleep.

I awoke in the morning refreshed, eager to meet the new day and ready for the adventures that awaited me. This was how every day should be for everyone — that grand feeling of arising with joy and anticipation. The birds were singing in the yard, celebrating their special place in the universal scheme of things. I stepped outside and took several deep breaths of the crisp, clear morning air, savoring the medley of honeysuckle, freshly mown grass and pine needles. These were the smells of my childhood. I looked forward to experiencing this new day, knowing it was bound to be filled with love and harmony.

~~~~~~~~~~~

Before long it was time to leave for the party. I drove through town and headed for the grange hall, enjoying familiar sights along the way. I hadn't told Doris I was coming. When she spotted me coming through the door, she let out something between a yelp and war whoop, and we rushed toward each other to embrace. Everyone loved Doris. As far back as I could remember, they always had. Growing up, she was that nice kid, the kind everyone wanted for a daughter. Her parents had known one of my dad's cousins in Colorado, where they all grew up, so the two families shared a common bond. Her birthday was a major celebration, and it seemed like half the county had shown up. I took a table with Tana, one of my former schoolmates, and her husband Ralph. Tana had taken the time to call me after my surgery, and I had not forgotten her kindness. We had some delectable chilled fruit and caught up on the past.

Several people took their turn at the microphone and presented their version of humorous events from Doris' life to the delight of the birthday child. A comedian had been hired for the occasion to spin an outrageous "Doris" yarn, and he had the audience rolling in the aisles. Eventually the party wound down, and I gathered my things to leave. Doris hugged me again and thanked me for coming, and she invited me to go to the fair with her later in the evening. We made plans to go for a late-afternoon swim and join in the festivities after dinner. June had told me to come and go as I pleased, knowing that I would enjoy visiting with some of my old friends.

Doris and her husband, Tom, lived south of town in an area filled with trees and teeming with wildlife. A swimming pool and a huge hot tub looked very inviting. We went for a swim first and then climbed into the warm, bubbling spa. If this didn't bring on a hot flash, nothing would. But to my surprise I felt nothing beyond the warmth of the water. Could it be the lowered stress level? I wondered. We relaxed for over an hour and then dressed to go to the Siskiyou County Fair. Simple pleasures, simple thrills — fine friends, childhood memories and a county fair. This was truly as good as it gets!

We strolled across the gravel parking lot and through one of the back gates to the fair. Why I still love this event is a mystery to me. Animal-rights supporters and county fairs don't really mix overly well. Maybe the carnival atmosphere, maybe the familiar faces and the sense of celebration all contribute to the mystical attraction. The smell of sawdust and lumber products and the sight of crowds of people in cowboy boots and western attire always gives me a natural high. Anyway, I don't have to understand it. I enjoy it, and that's all I need to know.

I hurried to the first booth selling hot, buttered corn and whipped out my wallet. The thought of butter dripping down my chin seemed almost too good to be decent. I love the way fresh corn squirts its sweet juices with wild abandon. As my teeth crunched into the first few rows of delicious golden kernels, I closed my eyes in ecstasy and thanked the universe for this simple joy.

As we moved through the crowds, familiar faces popped up everywhere. I passed several people I knew, and I stopped to chat. Others I thought I should know, so I nodded and smiled. The sky darkened, and hundreds of brilliant stars added their sparkle to the setting of the one and only Siskiyou County Fair. We visited and we ate; we went on rides and we laughed; we met old friends and we stayed and stayed late into the night. I had stepped out of my world of fear for a while and had enjoyed myself. I hoped some day this feeling would be permanent.

Long after I had let myself into my friends' home and hit the pillows, I heard Hooper slip in the back door. It was nearly two o'clock in the morning. Smiling in the dark, I pulled the sheet tightly around my neck and gave myself over to sleep, happily entering the land of dreams. That night my mind conjured up images resembling the patterns of an ever-changing kaleidoscope, where people and old haunts from days of long ago appeared in brilliant colors, separated and then returned in different dimensions.

Sunday morning we all went to church. I have long been a believer that what we may call coincidence is a universal connectedness and a part of our spiritual destiny. After having met June and Hooper in Portland, I discovered that they knew my family and even belonged to my home-town church. They had moved to Yreka from the Scott Valley area a few years after I'd left for college. We were all meant to know each other, and when the time was right, our paths crossed.

As the church began to fill up, several people stopped by to greet us warmly and inquire about my mother. Doris arrived and settled down next to me, still bubbling with the enjoyment of the previous day. Sitting on my left was Jewel Behnke, one of my favorite people in all of Siskiyou County. Jewel had been our choir director for many years and was my sixth-grade teacher at the Jackson Street Elementary School. I had blossomed in her classroom like a sunflower after the rain, nourished by her kindness and constant encouragement. Her husband, Warren, or "Pop," as he was called by his students, had been the music director for both Yreka schools. The entire family was wrapped up in music, and they were all warm, loving people.

The organ burst forth with several well-known hymns, and I basked in the pleasure of singing the alto line as I stood between my two friends. After the benediction, we joined the friendly, conversational hum of the traditional Methodist coffee hour. I was surprised how many people I still knew after so many years. And then a wonderful thing happened, which I will never forget. Jewel gave me a hug, and told me that she was very proud of what I had done with my life. The compliment came at a good time. I had recently been experiencing considerable guilt stemming from my inability to make life better for Mama. Having always been somewhat of a fixer, I was having difficulty accepting the fact that her life couldn't be fixed. I left the church wrapped in the warm afterglow of personal validation. Thank you, Jewel. Thank you for saying what I needed to hear.

~~~~~~~~~~

The following Monday my sentimental journey to paradise had come to an end. Leaving Yreka this time would be as difficult as refusing a piece of strawberry-rhubarb pie. Somehow I felt as though I were immersed for a time in my past, a past in which cancer had no place. But I had to return to Portland. I needed to be with Stan. The thought of being with my husband provided me with the necessary push to get into my car and finally, ever so slowly, turn the key. The motor engaged with a reassuring hum, and waving a wistful farewell to Hooper and June, I silently said good-bye to my quiet little town.

Between Medford and Rogue River I turned off the freeway and onto Old Highway 99. The familiar landmarks brought a smile to my heart. If Bobby's spirit had been close by in Yreka, the essence of Daryle Holt was everywhere here. Spotting her old house across the river, I slowed the car for a moment. I wondered who was spending their days on our river bank now and who closed their eyes in the dark of the night, listening to the rain beating rhythmically against the tin roof, in the place that once had been "my room."

Pulling back onto Interstate-5, I listened to Deepak Chopra's audio tape, *Ageless Body, Timeless Mind*. Since my bout with cancer, I had searched almost obsessively for things that might help me to avoid another *dance with death*. Dr. Chopra's books had become an integral part of my library. A few tapes, a few rest stops, and I arrived home.

I pulled into the driveway, got out of the car and walked toward the familiar blue house. The dogs barked their nonstop welcome behind the front door as I wrestled clumsily with my baggage and my key. Stan opened the door, and suddenly it felt good to be home. His low, resonant voice, now more than ever, was music to my soul. We had shared our lives for nearly thirty years now, and we had come to fit together like a pair of comfortable, well-worn shoes. I stayed in his hug for a long while, grateful for his steady gift of love and companionship.

Mama was seated at the dining room table peeling potatoes. She desperately wanted to keep busy, and we had created several little jobs that she could still manage, in the hope of boosting her waning self-esteem. She looked up and gave me a little half-smile. Had she not realized I'd been gone? An immediate flash of body heat reminded me of where I was and what had become my life. The Yreka party was definitely over now.

At times I felt like a stranger in my own body. Whoever said that life is never the same after breast cancer had hit upon the absolute truth. My visit in Yreka, the place of so many memories, had really driven it all home. There, I had fleetingly ventured into my past, returning to simpler, more secure times and feeling like the person I often feared I was losing. But now it was back to business, and a dry wind was beginning to parch my thirsting soul. Already I longed to return to greener pastures.

Often in the months that followed, I felt as though life was little more than treading water. My days were spent in the established humdrum, searching for answers—those elusive answers which, for the cancer patient, can never be found. Like a gerbil in its cage, furiously pedaling the wheel, I was running on a track that led to nowhere.

Always the same pitiful questions resurfaced: Why had this happened? Why? Was it my diet? Was it DDT? Was it the red meat I ate in my childhood? Could it have been Nutrasweet, the plums my neighbor had sprayed with defoliant? Or was it the estrogen I had been taking before my diagnosis—the estrogen that had made me feel like a sane, well-balanced human being instead of an unfocused Looney Tune? Then again, it could be my mind. I had always had an abnormal fear of cancer and had allowed thoughts of the disease to occupy my consciousness. Had I unknowingly invited it into my life? Maybe if Mama hadn't gotten sick, this wouldn't have happened? Maybe it was the stress of dealing with her dementia, the stress of losing my best friend. How could this possibly happen to me when there was no history of cancer in my family? Where had I gone haywire? What was the turning point? And the biggest question of all, pounding like a giant gong in my head: How could I keep it from happening again? What could I do?

Anger became an unwelcome emotion that constantly pervaded my life. Every time I strapped on my "breasts," I wanted to scream. I hated bras in the first place, and now they rubbed against the bullet-shaped drain hole, the unsightly, uncomfortable mess directly on what had once been the underside of my left breast. I tried sewing falsies into undershirts, but my entire chest would move as I turned from side to side. Much later I learned to pin the undershirt to my waistband to keep it from shifting. Part of the difficulty was having no one to blame, nowhere to direct my anger. I wanted someone or something to hate.

Sometimes it wasn't so difficult. I hated the women in the Victoria's Secret catalogues that arrived weekly in our mailbox. And I hated the men who were aroused by the perfect bodies that graced every full-color page. If I even suspected that Stan was looking at a female, I attempted to assess the direction of his glance. What was he thinking? Did the pitiful sight of my disfigured chest evoke fantasies of romantic interludes with "real" women? My emotions were so close to the surface that the slightest inconsequential event would bring on a teary outburst. I didn't like this stranger I had become, but I was at a loss how to get rid of her.

Summer was over before I knew it, and I was determined to have a better year than the previous one. At school, there was a new teacher and new programs, both of which I considered an opportunity to start fresh. I would write myself reminders. I would listen intently. I WOULD FOCUS. For the most part, work seemed considerably better. Some of my self-confidence was beginning to return. Work became my refuge from the depressing atmosphere of the home front.

In an attempt to create a new me, I decided to change the way I wore my hair. I had worn short hair for ten years— just about the estimated age of my tumor. Maybe that was it! Maybe short hair caused cancer. Maybe if I let my hair grow to my waist, my breasts would grow back.

There I went again! Like a dog with his favorite bone, I couldn't resist bringing the subject of cancer into everything I did, ate, drank or dreamed—past and present. I was fanatically occupied with thoughts of *cancer this, cancer that, cancer everything.* When would I stop? When would I stop replaying that same old tape, allowing this killer to define my life? Or, as a friend of mine suggested emphatically: "Get out of your box."

At this point the idea of reconstructive surgery became more and more appealing. I had heard that there were two different types of procedures available. The first, and easiest by far, involved saline implants. My only objection was the use of a silicone sheath. An acquaintance of mine had suffered for many years as an apparent result of silicone implants. She had experienced a variety of problems, endured considerable pain and had even tested positive for lupus. The idea of silicone in my body frightened me.

The second procedure involved transplanting fat and muscle from the abdominal area. I liked the idea of using my own tissue and having a much-needed tummy tuck. Many women experience weight gain on Tamoxifen, and I was no exception. What was left of my body was becoming Rubenesque, and I disliked it intensely. Having been a dancer, I had come to attach undue importance to my physical attributes. Life has a way of teaching us lessons, but I was fighting the learning process every step of the way. Being disfigured was depressing enough. I entertained the idea of building bigger and better breasts. Dolly Parton, move over!

At one of the hospitals, before-and-after photos of reconstructive surgery were available, so Stan and I decided to check it out. In the pictures the breasts looked pretty good, but the nipples, for the most part, looked unnatural.

Ever the cynic, I considered the fact that these pictures must surely represent the best work of each surgeon. I wondered what their bloopers looked like? I had read somewhere that when consulting a plastic surgeon, one should ask to see photos of the best and worst results. Yeah, right! I could just see some surgeon whipping out an eight-by-ten of some poor woman with her breasts off-center and then asking when you wanted to schedule your surgery. Stan and I left the photo exhibit feeling rather ambivalent. The one thing I did know for certain was that this was not the right time for me to make a final decision. I just wasn't ready.

Life went on in my strange new world. Two positive events were noted on my fall agenda: the *Survivors' Luncheon* and the 1995 *Race for the Cure*. The Survivors' Luncheon was held on the Saturday preceding the race. I had arranged to meet Darlene and some of her friends, and we took our places at a round table with several other women. Soon the room was packed. Breast cancer survivors were wearing pink carnations, while their guests had been given white ones.

Five of the women at our table were survivors. The woman sitting on my right had undergone two modified radicals six years apart, both for carcinoma. She had opted for reconstructive surgery of the TRAM flap (tummy tuck) variety and was quite satisfied with the results. The only problem, she said, was the loss of abdominal muscles. She could no longer do sit-ups and had to use her arms to bring herself to a sitting position. That fact would be a problem for me. My job involved lifting students, and I was already seeing a chiropractor for back trouble. The abdominal muscles are important in supporting the back, and the possible effect from their loss was of some concern to me.

As I looked around the crowded room, I wondered how many of us would be alive next year. Behind every pink carnation was a life in jeopardy, a story that might be approaching its final chapter. We had all stared death in the face. Someone had written or said that breast cancer was a valuable experience, an experience that changed our lives for the better and taught us many important lessons. About all it had taught me so far was that I wanted no part of it ever again.

The special luncheon speaker asked for a show of hands for one, two, five and ten-year- and-more survivors. With each increase of years, the show of hands became smaller and smaller. One woman at our table had made it for twenty-five years. Surely she must be cured. I hoped I was.

The *Race for the Cure* was held the following day. I didn't feel up to running and had signed up to walk. Sue Ripley, one of my friends from our church choir had volunteered to walk with me. We gathered on a hazy September morning at Tom McCall Waterfront Park in downtown Portland. Some people had formed teams with members from various businesses, and others were joined by friends and family. A young girl passed by with a sign on her back revealing that she was racing for the cure in memory of her mother. In the lower right corner of her shirt was a picture of a young woman—the mother she had lost to this *serial killer*. My sign was in memory of my two aunts, Ruby and Dorothy Needles. Cancer had claimed my Aunt Dorothy less than a month after we lost Aunt Ruby.

All around me were testimonials to the power of human love and to the senseless grief and devastation brought on by this age-old killer disease for which there is still no known cure. The pictures of loved ones on display drove home more than ever the fact that these were real people, not statistics. These women had lived and loved. They had left behind their husbands, children, friends and lovers, never again to experience life's tender moments. They did not ask for this.

The crowd stretched into the distance as far as I could see. The moving mass of dedicated humanity was accented by bright-pink visors. What a powerful statement those pink visors! There we were, all of us, fighting for our lives, hoping to live another year, desperately wishing that someone, somewhere, would find a cure and give us back our peace of mind. Just as the speakers and performers had empowered us at the luncheon, the sheer numbers of devoted racers were leaving their mark here. I felt love in my heart for every last one of them.

I looked around for Darlene. Finding anyone in the crowd was hopeless. We had planned to meet here, but we had forgotten to name an exact spot. Sue and I finished walking and, caught up in the spirit of the day, decided to walk home. That was a big mistake for me. Every joint and muscle in my body cried out for rest by the time we crossed the Ross Island Bridge to the east side of the city. We still had a mile or so to go, and I was determined to persevere. My clothing was wet and clammy, and my two prostheses felt like water-filled balloons. But it had been a good day, a day of gathering strength and solidarity. When the figures were in, 18,201 people had drawn together for a common cause. What a grand cause—The Race for the Cure.

More dead than alive, I stumbled into the house, peeled off my sweaty clothing and poured myself a tall glass of sun tea. I stepped out onto the deck where a lounge chair beckoned with promises of rest. I collapsed in content exhaustion, closed my eyes and let the cool breeze brush my hot face. When I opened my eyes again, night had fallen.

~~~~~~~~~~

By October, my life was beginning to fall back into place. Occasionally I even felt a bit like my old self. After making my yearly appointment for a pelvic exam, I thought I noticed a drop of blood in the toilet. The examination proved uneventful, but my doctor decided an endometrial biopsy was in order. After all, good old Tamoxifen could cause uterine cancer. The last time I'd undergone one of these cheery little procedures, I'd practically found myself hanging from the light fixture. After listening to a few minutes of my whining and snivelling, my doctor arranged for the appointment to include a pericervical block. The injections at the edge of my cervix were somewhat uncomfortable, but they effectively blocked out the more agonizing pain. The results of the test were negative. I had been certain they would be. I now had one less phantom in my life.

~~~~~~~~~~

Time marches on, as they say, and soon the year had come and gone. It was spring again! One night in May, I was routinely running my fingers over my bony chest. Something felt weird. My fingers stopped at a small, hard lump. For some reason, I didn't panic, but I did make an appointment with the surgeon who had removed my right breast.

My doctor carefully examined the area for a while until she located the spot which was no bigger than a beebee. She was confident that it was nothing serious, but she also understood my need to know for sure. She recommended we do a biopsy in her office. What with the relative numbness of my chest, the pain would be negligible. WRONG! She deadened the area with local anesthesia. I could watch the whole procedure in the reflection of the windowpane. As the scalpel sliced away, I tensed my muscles and grimaced.

"Is that pain or pressure?" she asked.

"That's pain," I managed to utter between clenched teeth.

"Better give it another shot."

Finally it was over, and she showed me what she had removed. She would send the tissue to the lab, but she was certain that it was benign. She carefully closed the incision, and I was on my way. The biopsy report was negative. The bump had been nothing more than a nerve bundle. No wonder it had hurt like hell. After that I stopped feeling around my chest so often. Maybe I was beginning to trust my body.

After a year and a half of strapping on my boobs every time I left the house, I started to go running in just a T-shirt. After all, we seldom saw anyone we knew, and what did I care what strangers thought? The choice was between my comfort and theirs. This was, after all, only a matter of perception. The time had come to start reclaiming my body. Once in a while my self-consciousness surfaced, and I would stuff my chest pockets with cotton balls. But ultimately I was feeling better about myself.

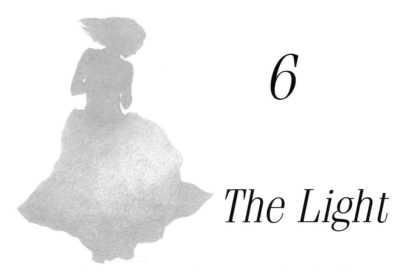

6

The Light

*"We must be willing to get rid of the life
we've planned so as to have
the life that is waiting for us."*

—Joseph Campbell

Healing arrived gradually, slipping into my life in a subtle aura of heightened awareness. The call of the red-winged blackbird and the whisper of the wind in the tall trees awakened a place deep in my spirit, a place I had feared was forever lost. With the passage of time, my heart began to dance, and the good days finally outnumbered the bad. One morning I was standing in the kitchen brewing a pot of green tea when I had an epiphany. I realized that I had actually crawled out of bed without experiencing the sudden shock wave of remembrance that every morning had jolted me into the stark realization that I was now a *cancer patient*. Thoughts of the "Big C" had not occupied their usual place in my first waking moments. Could it be that the devastating events of the last two years were   finally losing some of their depraved power? This was a milestone of sorts.

As the days went on, I was more and more grateful for my new friend Alyce. Always there for me, she spoke with the voice of one who had lived the experience, giving credence to my feelings. But this year, three-and-a-half years after her surgery, she was more relaxed, and I wanted some of what she had found for herself. We were standing in the hall talking one day about the fears and the uncertainties that come with a breast cancer diagnosis.

Her words were like a gift from an angel: "I remember sitting at the table trembling, my mind frozen by fear — out of control. My husband didn't know what to do for me. Finally, that day I made a conscious decision. I decided I just wasn't going to live my life that way. This wasn't really living. I had a wonderful husband and a family I wanted to enjoy. I had grandchildren I wanted to lavish with love. I was grateful for everything. My fears were destroying everything, and they had to be banished. It was high time!"

That conversation proved to be one of my turning points. If Alyce had done it, so could I—I could reclaim my life. As Louise Hay so succinctly puts it, "All you have to do is think a thought." My thoughts were mine, mine to change.

I had turned the corner. Instead of listening to talk shows after work, I rested quietly and focused on guided meditations. Every aspect of my life would undergo scrutiny. I would reexamine everything for positive or negative input. Even the daily ritual of reading my mail would undergo a transformation. I discarded negative, fear-evoking letters from animal-rights groups and kept only the remittance envelopes. No more horrible stories. My mind would be filled instead with thoughts of animals safe in loving homes or in guarded sanctuaries. Helping financially didn't necessitate reading the ugly details. Positive thoughts breed positive attitudes. Positive attitudes breed healing of body, mind and soul.

Feeling the need for acquiring more wellness tools, I entertained the idea of looking for a support group. I had purposely avoided any involvement with such groups after my surgeries, fearing that the stories of other women in various stages of the disease would literally scare me to death. Surely someone must have a group focusing on the mind-body connection, focusing on the positive. I would seek out someone with a holistic approach.

"Seek and ye shall find!" I was reading *The Bridge*, the local newsletter from *A Course in Miracles*. The words of an advertisement fairly jumped off the page: THE HEALING PLACE. I headed straight for the telephone. The woman's voice on the other end of the line conveyed the exact feeling I was looking for. This was my answer. She told me that the next session would be held in two weeks. Would I be there? Absolutely. I could hardly wait.

The day finally arrived, and I drove across town to The Healing Place. The building, an inviting older home with hardwood floors and a little fountain in one corner, felt comfortable from the moment I walked inside. Something was baking in the kitchen. The facilitator, Judy Allen, met me in the front hall. She had dealt with a breast cancer recurrence and had successfully beaten the odds. This gentle woman exuded a genuine quality and a remarkable depth of character. She knew what she was all about, and it showed.

Comfortable chairs and an assortment of pillows were arranged in a circle in the living room where we would meet for four hours. A stack of books sat on a table, one of which caught my immediate attention. The title was something on the order of Five Thousand Spontaneous Remissions. This was my kind of stuff. Based on her own experience with breast cancer, Judy had published her own book entitled *The Five Stages of Getting Well*. The title was set in firm juxtaposition to the five stages of death and dying outlined by Elizabeth Kubler-Ross in her well known book, *On Death and Dying.*

The four-hour session flew by like the wind, ending with a guided meditation. Before I left, I picked up a copy of Judy's book. Walking quietly to my car, I could sense a slight shift in perception. I hoped it would be permanent.

A full week passed before I found adequate time to devote myself to reading *The Five Stages of Getting Well.* But as soon as I started reading, I was mesmerized and devoured the entire contents. The author spoke of having discovered "a joyful alternative to dying and death." The impact of her message was so strong that after I finished the last page, I went upstairs to my desk and pulled out my "Breast Cancer" file. Without a second thought, I carried it outside to the garbage can. Lifting the lid, I dropped the folder unceremoniously into the foul-smelling heap of trash. The muffled thud carried with it a much-needed and welcome finality. I had dropped a great deal of my cancer load right into the garbage. That was where it belonged. Case closed. I'd get on with life.

Lightheartedly, I turned my back on the dented trash can and reflected on the countless hours I had spent poring over my pathology report, reading and digesting every word, over and over again. How much power had I given to this despicable disease? How much fear had I allowed to poison my unconscious mind?

Once inside the house, I pulled out a crisp new file folder and slowly wrote the word, "Healing" in prominent letters across the tab. Nothing dramatic. No fireworks. Just a long-over-due closure. Thank you, Judy. I sat for a while at my desk absorbed in the contentment of the moment.

A wise man once said, *"If someone did to us what we do to ourselves, we'd take out a gun and shoot him."* I had been on a path to destruction and on my way to spiritual and emotional suicide. We can do that, or we can choose to do as author, Shawna Schuh, prescribes in her book, *51 Ways To Pick Up Your Get-Up and Go.* We can pick ourselves up and get going. I knew I could make it back to where I had been before. I could become the old Rachael again *and then some.* By then I knew with unerring certainty that if I failed to make some changes, I'd eventually have a recurrence.

Another stepping stone on my path to recovery was my decision to have some counseling sessions. Despite the meas-urable progress in some areas of my life, one stress factor was constant. I couldn't escape the slow but sure process of losing my mother—little by little, day by day. I watched helplessly as this sweet, tortured little soul struggled to cling to the last few vestiges of her dignity. Her face remained lovely, not unlike that of a delicate porcelain doll, but her eyes had become dull and puzzled as she strove in vain to untangle the increasingly confusing world around her.

Simple tasks such as putting a stamp on an envelope and addressing it, had become arduous and finally impossible. One by one, I stopped giving her those little jobs, as her frustration grew and her self-worth waned. When the tasks disappeared, time hung heavily on her hands. Every day she looked sadder, and try as I would, I just couldn't make it better. I could provide love and care, but I couldn't unlock her mind and restore her reasoning abilities. She looked at me one day and said she felt as though she were living in a cloud, and she couldn't understand why she had to keep waking up.

"I've lived a good life, but the good part is over, and I wish I could just drift away and be done with it." She was having one of her more lucid moments. I sat on the floor next to her, stroking her hand, knowing that she desperately needed someone to validate her feelings.

"I understand, Mama," I replied with a heavy heart. "I'd probably feel the same way. I'm so sorry this is happening to you. I love you, and I'd do anything in the world to make you happy."

Her eyes strayed somewhere above my head into the distance, as she asked, "What have I done to offend my Maker that He would do this to me?"

I took her in my arms and held her close, so close I could feel her failing heart as it struggled with its erratic beat. As I stroked her white hair, we cried together.

"You didn't do anything, Mama. It's just a disease. It just happens sometimes. God doesn't do it."

But in my heart of hearts, I wondered why He didn't stop it. One of her favorite prayers had always been, "Father, let us radiate the light of Your eternal truth into every life we touch." For her, those lives had been many. She'd always been faithful to her chosen task. So where was the mercy she deserved? In my childlike anguish, I was becoming increasingly resentful of this lack of rightfully earned Divine intervention. Try as I would, I couldn't shake that feeling.

Finally I telephoned my doctor and requested a referral to a social worker. My issues with cancer and caregiving were simply too much for me to handle without help. Dr. M. understood my needs and gave me the name of a woman in Portland's elegant northwest hills. I made an appointment the same day.

The sloping and curving street of the west hills was lined with stately elm trees, so tall that their branches fairly disappeared into the sky. Sunlight filtered through the shimmering leaves as they danced lightly in the breeze, making ever-changing patterns on the shiny hood of my car. Lingering pensively, I took in bits of the verdant energy around me. A beautiful building of classic architecture loomed directly to my right. This was the place.

Jean, the counselor I was to see, had her office on the third floor. A magnificent wooden staircase, an opulent masterpiece reminiscent of Scarlet O'Hara's Tara, flowed upward from the center of the main floor. I tried to envision what might await me. Would I lie on a couch and spill my guts and feel better because I could pay someone to let me dump a load of misery? Why am I always so cynical when I'm about to experience something new which has not as yet earned my seal of approval?

Puffing my way up to the third-floor waiting room, I paused and took a few deep breaths. I settled myself in a chair, reached for a magazine and waited. I was a few minutes early.

At precisely four o'clock, the door to the counselor's inner sanctum opened and a smiling woman with dark hair and a friendly, round face called my name. I had imagined encountering a thin-lipped, scrawny person in a tailored suit, a silk blouse and a two-hundred-dollar pair of Charles Jourdan shoes. Jean was a pleasant surprise. She was dressed comfortably in a softly flowing blue skirt, a loose-fitting blouse and a pair of casual flats. I sensed in her a sincerity, coupled with a genuine caring that put me at ease immediately.

She listened attentively to what I had to say, asking very few questions, letting me take the lead. I made my next appointment and left with the feeling of having started something necessary, yet at the same time comfortable. I looked forward to my next session.

As the weeks passed, Jean obtained an overview of what she was hearing from my rambling. I felt completely at ease in the atmosphere of absolute safety she provided for her clients, and my eyes were opened to the fact that it was okay that I couldn't fix everything. I finally "got it" that sadness, anger and frustration were normal reactions, natural responses to difficult circumstances. The counseling sessions with Jean were both energizing and at the same time soothing, not unlike a hot bath after a long, hard day.

~~~~~~~~~~

It was a lovely morning that summer of 1996. I went to Mother's room to wake her for breakfast. As I opened the door, I saw her lying on the floor, soaking in urine. Even though Stan and I had a monitor in our room, we hadn't heard her fall. Kneeling beside her on the floor, I questioned her gently: "Honey, how did you fall?"

"Did I fall?" she asked, her voice registering surprise.

"Mom, you're on the floor. What happened?"

"I'm on the floor?" Again surprised.

I yelled for Stan. Together we helped her to the side of the bed.

In order to remove her wet clothes, we asked her to stand up, but her mind couldn't process what we were saying, and she remained seated. Just about then I was having a major hot flash and wanted to scream. We finally managed to get her to a chair, and I sponged her off and managed to change her into dry clothes. Supported by Stan on one side and by me on the other, she managed to walk to the living room couch. I went into the kitchen and poured myself a cup of green tea. Stan was leaning against the counter, visibly shaken. Overcome by exhaustion, I felt myself slipping out of control.

"Stan, I just can't do this anymore. I just can't!" My voice broke, and I collapsed into a chair. Stan nodded in silent agreement. We spent the rest of the evening avoiding conversation about the inevitable. I woke up the next morning dreading the chore that lay ahead of me, which I knew must be done. So began the unhappy business of searching for a decent adult foster-care home.

Fortunately, I was still seeing Jean at the time. Slumping down into one of the low-slung chairs in her office, I recounted the latest events. For the first time since I had gone into therapy, I reached for a Kleenex.

"I'm sorry. I think I'm losing it," I mumbled between tears.

"It's okay to cry. That's what the tissue is for."

I went on with my sad story while Jean listened patiently. Finally she spoke. "I think it's very good that you knew when you couldn't go on taking care of your mother. That's healthy. I'd venture to say that two months ago you couldn't have made that decision."

Up to that moment I'd felt like a failure. How could I put my mother in the home of a stranger? Who would love her as I did? Who would hug her and tuck her in at night? What was wrong with me that I couldn't take it any more?

Suddenly my mind shifted. Putting my mother into the hands of a caregiver would not be easy, but it had to be done. Besides my own emotional well-being, I had Stan to consider. His diabetes had shot out of control lately, and our relationship had become strained. Being torn between the two people I so dearly loved was fracturing my sanity.

Another thing that helped me to persevere was something Mama had told me over and over during the years I was growing up. She had always said not to feel badly if the time ever came when I needed to "put her somewhere." She realized that I had no siblings to help shoulder the responsibility if she became infirm. What would she say if she were in her right mind? I knew the answer.

I prayed, and we searched for the perfect place for my mother. Most of the homes we inspected were beautifully furnished and spotless, but none of their operators portrayed the sort of person I would consider entrusting with the care of a loved one. Elder care was obviously a business for these people, nothing more, nothing less. My heart sank lower and lower as I walked in and out of the well-groomed, highly polished adult foster homes.

Blessings upon blessings! Finally, there she was—the perfect caregiver. Her name was Grace, and she floated gently into our lives one Saturday afternoon when I was truly at my wits' end. I had been sitting on the couch praying. Feeling the need to blow off the mounting steam of my frustration, I called Peggy, one of my friends from work. Her father had died a few months ago, and I had often heard her talk about his loving caregiver, Grace. I remembered hearing that Grace had prayed with him and gently eased his passing. The only reason I hadn't attempted to locate her before was that I thought she was too far away, too far for a daily visit with Mama after a full day's work at school.

"Do you want me to call Grace?" Peggy took the lead.

"Isn't she way out in east county?"

"No, her place is on 128th and Raymond."

"That's not so far," I admitted.

"I don't know whether she has a vacancy, but if she doesn't, she might know someone."

"Could you find out? I don't know where to turn."

I hung up the phone and walked out onto the deck with a tall glass of iced tea. A few minutes later, the phone rang. It was Peggy.

"I have wonderful news for you. Grace has an opening coming up in two weeks, and she will take your mom. You'll love her."

Finding Grace turned out to be a gift from God. That evening we asked Margaret to stay with Mama while we drove to *Stillwater Guest Home,* aptly named for the twenty-third Psalm. Grace, a kind, gentle and gracious woman opened the door and welcomed us into her home. And it was truly a home and not a facility.

In the spacious living room, a perky wisp of a woman sat knitting on the couch. We found out that her name was Emma, and she was ninety-eight years old. Grace settled herself in a comfortable-looking overstuffed chair across from the sofa.

"Sit down. Tell me about your mother." Grace looked at us with an inviting smile.

I talked for a while about Mama's condition and her needs and expressed my concerns. "She's my mother. I love her. I want her to be surrounded with love. She needs to be hugged. She needs someone to pray with her and care about her."

Grace's eyes brightened. "I hug all my ladies, and I'd love to pray with her if she'll let me."

"She'll let you," I replied happily. "She's a preacher's kid. She can still read, but she doesn't remember what she has read. Reading her devotions to other people gives her a sense of purpose. She needs to feel valued."

"We can do that. We'll do it every day at the table." I knew she meant what she said. I felt as though the weight of the world had been lifted off my shoulders. If I had to place my mother in someone else's care, it would have to be someone like Grace. Grace! How aptly she was named—Grace. Everything about this woman and her home felt right. Peggy had been right. Grace informed us that she would have an opening in two weeks.

As gently as I could, I prepared Mama for what lay ahead—change. To my surprise, she was very understanding about the impending move. We explained that I had to go back to work in the fall and that Stan just couldn't handle her care. She put her tiny, age-worn hand on my forearm. "You always know what to do. I'm sure you've made the right decision." At that moment she was, fairly clear. She no longer remembered my name or understood the mother/daughter relationship, but she seemed to know that I loved her, whoever I was.

Two weeks later, on a sunny August day, we helped my mother into the car and drove her to her new home. Grace was watching for us and met us outside. She put her arm around Mama and introduced herself. As we all crossed the threshold, she looked at my little angel and took her hand.

"Welcome to my home. I'm so happy to have you. Come in and meet Emma."

Mama settled herself comfortably on a blue, fluffy couch, and I sat down beside her. I wondered if she would think it was the blue couch in our living room where she had spent so much time during the last few months. Grace spoke to her in a soft, soothing voice, and I could tell that their spirits were already touching. She told Mama that she needed someone to read the devotions and say the blessings at dinner. For the first time in many months, I could see my mother's eyes brighten, even taking on a bit of their old familiar light. Stan caught my eye across the room, and I knew he was seeing the same thing. This had been a guided decision. God was in this room, and all was well.

When we left Mama's new home, she was stretched out on the living room couch with her feet up. She looked relaxed and perfectly content to be where she was. Maybe she didn't even realize she had moved. I didn't know how to feel.

We were on our way home, just the two of us. We could stop off anywhere we liked for as long as we liked. For once, we didn't have to hurry home. "Let's go to lunch," I suggested after a few blocks of silence. Stan seemed pleased about having lunch out and looked around for a restaurant.

We stopped at a Thai restaurant and savored the fragrant morsels of a stir-fry meal, knowing that we could stay as long as we wanted, and Mama would be safe. I looked at my husband across the table. Stan's face had already begun to relax. He looked ten years younger. Even his voice sounded different when he asked, "Do you want to run tonight?" looking at me expectantly.

I thought for a moment. We *could* run again. We could run down by the river and afterwards sit in the moonlight with no thoughts of rushing home— no urgency. We could flow with our own needs for a change, pamper ourselves with leisure time and take care of each other. At the risk of sounding selfish, I was relieved. I loved my mother, but my love no longer reached her. I could feel my tension slowly dissolving. There's a time and a season for everything. The time had come for Stan and me to do some catching up. It was our season.

That evening we decided to take our meals on the deck for a while. Mama's favorite time of day had been the evening meal. She loved sitting around the table as part of the family. Though she usually only wanted cream soups and mocha, she always commented on the wonderful food and how pretty the table looked. Sitting next to her empty place would be too much to handle for a while.

We ate on the deck until the late fall weather drove us indoors. I had visited Mama daily for two months and watched her enjoy her soup at Grace's table. Emma was always at her side, prompting her to eat and talking into her good ear. I was satisfied I had done the right thing. I was thrilled that the change was working out for all three of us. Mother was safe; she was content. Stan and I enjoyed being alone again. Fall was gone before we knew it, and the chill of winter filled the air.

Miracle upon miracles! For three whole days during the holiday season, Mama knew me. She recognized me. After so many months, she said my name, and it gave me, if only for a short time, a sense of having her back. Having no siblings, I often felt as though my entire history was disappearing into some nebulous never-never land, that far-off place that housed my mother's memory of who I was, who we were.

For three days I was someone's daughter again. My God, how I'd missed that—missed her! And then she was gone again, retreating to that place where I could not follow and where only her spirit held the answers.

Barbara gave me an insight one day while we chatted over a holiday lunch at one of our favorite restaurants. She said that knowing me and calling me by my name was Mama's Christmas present to me. It made sense. It was true. This had been a message from her spirit to mine. Perhaps it went something like this:

"I love you, and I haven't forgotten you. And long after our world ceases to exist, I will still love you, for God gave you to me. We will always be together."

That love is mine to keep...always.

By the end of January, Mama began asking to stay in bed. I visited her regularly and one day, Grace met me at the door, her face wistful, her eyes sad. "If you have anything you want to say to her, you should probably do it now," she said softly as she reached for my hands.

"Your mother has almost stopped eating, and the nurse says that it won't be long now."

I leaned over the bed and studied the tiny figure nearly lost in the mound of covers. Her eyes were open, and she reached up and touched my face in a loving gesture, trying to say something. I couldn't make it out. She seemed to be repeating the same thing over and over, but it sounded like gibberish.

I leaned in closer to her and began talking to her. "Mom, I want you to know that you've been the best mother anyone could ever have. You have given me everything I'll ever need. You gave me a sense of values, and you taught me about God. I always knew you loved me, no matter how often I messed up. I'll miss you, Mom, but I know you're tired, and it's okay to go whenever you're ready."

I kissed her forehead and remained quietly at her bedside. Her eyes were closed, and her breathing was labored. What was keeping her alive? What kept her tired little heart beating? Finally, I left the room.

For the next few days amazing Grace worked her magic, singing *Jesus Loves Me* and playing tapes of old familiar hymns in my mother's room. She would stroke Mama's head and tell her that pretty soon Jesus would come and make her well. What an outpouring of love and caring. We were truly blessed when Grace came into our lives. We will be grateful to her forever.

On February 7, 1997, my angel finally got her wings. I like to believe that she floated into the light and took my father's hand. Wherever she is, I'm sure she's with God, and I'm sure she's at peace.

At long last, my peace has also come to pass... that sweet, serene peace that comes with the knowledge that Mama is free and no longer in pain. Her presence is everywhere, and in my heart I know that she wants me to be happy and go on with my life. One of the things I found among her papers was a letter, handwritten on a steno pad:

> *My Darling Daughter, Rachael,*
>
>   *When I am gone, don't grieve for me. Just think of me often and know that I have had a wonderful life, remarkably free of illness. I have enjoyed the love and respect of my family, tender care from you and Stan, and more blessings that I can enumerate. I am trying to make my transition as easy as possible for you. You and Stan will always have my love, wherever you are, and I hope both of you will always be happy.*
>
>   *Love,*
>
>   *Mom*

The letter was followed by the details I would need to close her estate. How many mothers leave their daughters with a gift of such beauty? I have been blessed beyond measure. My tribute to this wonderful woman is to carry on her life through the living of mine. Because of her love, I can stand tall in the face of adversity.

The remainder of my days will be spent as a breast cancer activist, helping to raise public awareness and fighting for dollars to fund research and education.

This book is my first step. A portion of the proceeds will be donated to *Global Walk,* the monumental undertaking of Polly Letofsky, a young woman who is currently walking world-wide, in an effort to raise funds for breast cancer awareness and education.* As long as anyone will listen, I will tell my story.

No woman should be faced with the prospect of forfeiting her life to this murderous intruder that hides silently in the sanctity of her breast, undetected until it is so often too late. No woman should face the trauma of disfigurement or the sleep-less nights wrought with fear of a fatal recurrence. We need a cure and we needed it yesterday. As the saying goes: "We can run, but we can't hide." So we must stand up and fight.

Rachael Clearwater

*http://www.globalwalk.org

7

20/20 Hindsight
Dos and Donts and Helpful Hints

"The meaningful question is never what we did yesterday but what we have learned from it and are doing today."

— Marianne Williamson

Mammography

I can't say enough about mammography, because I literally owe my life to this procedure. My tumor was detected before my surgeon could find it during his examination. By then the malignant growth was approximately two centimeters in diameter and had, in all probability, been growing for more than eight years. Many tumors are buried deep within the breast and can only be detected through mammography. Had I not coasted past the proper date for this annual procedure, my prognosis would undoubtedly be somewhat better. Had I neglected to go at all, I would be well on my way to pushing up daisies.

A mammogram is simply an X-ray of the breast. It is not one-hundred-percent effective, but it is extremely valuable, especially for post-menopausal women whose breast tissue has lost a considerable degree of density. The radiation risk is negligible, and the procedure is simple. I am convinced that every woman over the age of forty owes herself an annual mammogram. Money simply is not an issue. Free mammograms are available at various places at different times. For further information, call the Komen Foundation hotline: 1-800-404-8241. And even if you must go into debt in order to pay for a mammogram, the cost certainly beats dying.

Ultrasound

If anything questionable shows up on your mammogram, your doctor may suggest that you have an ultrasound done. Do it. You may be able to put your mind at ease immediately. The procedure utilizes high-frequency sound waves and is totally painless and non-intrusive. A gel is applied to the breast, and an instrument, called a transducer, is run over the problem area. An image on a computer screen tells the technician whether the targeted mass is solid or fluid-filled. Tumors are solid. Harmless cysts often contain fluid. The ultrasound approach is particularly useful for women with dense, hard-to-read breast tissue. No radiation is involved.

Needle Biopsy

If you have an inconclusive mammogram, and for some reason your doctor doesn't recommend an excisional (surgical) biopsy, you may want to inquire about a needle biopsy. It is easy, relatively painless, and potentially lifesaving. I was diagnosed three years later than I should have been, because a surgeon decided against this procedure after my doctor had recommended it. Those three years of delay could have cost me my life. At the very least my prognosis deteriorated. Don't play around with your life.

Surgical Options

Get educated before you get cut. If a surgeon suggests a mastectomy, ask why. If you're not satisfied, insist on a second or third opinion. If you are timid about questioning your surgeon, or think he might be insulted—stop! Think about your own feelings. After all, surgeons get over it, but you have to live with yourself and your decisions. Your relationship with yourself is certainly more important than your relationship with your doctor. You can always find a new doctor. Remember that members of the medical profession are paid by you and your insurance company. This makes them, in effect, your employees.

Sutures

When surgery is required, insist that your doctor use subcutaneous sutures. If he refuses to do so, dump him or insist on a plastic surgeon to do the job. The scars from the staples on my left side have stretched — some to a length of an eighth of an inch. They're ugly, and they were unnecessary. No one told me that I would be stapled, or I would have been horrified.

Nerve Preservation

One possible effect of removing lymph nodes for dissection may be numbness in the armpit and along the inside of the upper arm. This happens when the nerves lying in the surgical field are cut. According to Dr. Susan Love, the nerves are difficult, but not always impossible to save. Tell your surgeon that the sensation in your arm is important to you and that you want every effort made to preserve the nerves. Shaving a numb armpit is no fun.

I hope that much of the agony of multiple lymph-node dissection will soon be a thing of the past. Studies are currently being carried out to determine whether removal of the sentinel, or first, lymph node in a cluster can conclusively foretell the presence or absence of cancer in the entire node group.

Endometrial Biopsy

One of the possible side effects of the medication Tamoxifen is endometrial cancer. Although the percentages are very low, some doctors recommend an annual uterine biopsy just to be safe. The procedure is quite painful, but much of the intense pain can be alleviated with the application of a pericervical block (injections around the cervix to block the pain). This method of blocking out pain has worked extremely well for me, and I would recommend it for anyone with a low-to-moderate pain threshold.

Copies of Reports

You have the right to obtain your medical information. Your doctor or surgeon should be willing to provide you with a copy of your pathology, radiology and other reports upon request and explain everything to you point by point. I know of at least one case in which annual follow-up was recommended, but the patient was never advised. This particular woman saw no urgency and, being under fifty, felt safe in waiting three years to have another mammogram. When she finally did go to mammography, a biopsy was performed immediately, and a large, aggressive, malignant tumor came to light.

Patient-Controlled Analgesic (P.C.A.)

P.C.A. is an extremely empowering tool for the surgical patient and is available upon request at most hospitals. It allows the patient to push a button and access the prescribed pain killer rather than to wait for an injection from a busy nurse. Only a specified amount of analgesic will be released, eliminating the possibility of an overdose. Patient Controlled Analgesic is helpful in relieving pain anxiety.

Drains

Insist that drains must be exited below the bra line. I can't stress this enough. The first thing I do when I come into my house is rip off my bra with the prostheses because of the continual discomfort caused by one of my drain scars. The scar is the size and shape of a bullet hole, and is more than annoyingly uncomfortable under the pressure of a bra.

Adjuvant Therapy

The decisions regarding chemotherapy, hormone therapy,

radiation and other treatments are of paramount importance. Consult at least three professionals. Don't trust one person with your life. You're too important.

Reading

First read to get educated. You can't afford to be ignorant where your life is concerned. Gather vital information as soon after your diagnosis as possible. If you pick up a copy of *Dr. Susan Love's Breast Book,* you'll get a sound education on the subject. After that, move on to books which deal in a positive way with breast cancer and offer hope and courage. One of my big mistakes was to continue to read everything I could find on the subject of breast cancer for nearly a year following my diagnosis. Looking back, I can see that I undoubtedly added unnecessarily to my level of anxiety and reinforced my fears.

Some of the books I found helpful are:

Anatomy of an Illness, (1979) Norman Cousins, Norton, N.Y.

Head First, (1989) Norman Cousins, E.P. Dutton, N.Y.

Love, Medicine and Miracles, (1986) Bernie Siegel, M.D., Harper & Row, N.Y.

Peace, Love and Healing, (1986) Bernie Siegel, M.D., Harper & Row, N.Y.

Quantum Healing, (1989) Deepak Chopra, M.D., Bantam Books, N.Y.

The Five Stages of Getting Well, (1992) Judy Edwards Allen, Ph.D., Lifetime Publishing, Portland, OR.

Choices in Healing, (1992) Michael Lerner, The MIT Press, Cambridge, Mass.

Ageless Body, Timeless Mind, 1993) Deepak Chopra, M.D, Random House, Inc., N.Y.

Beating Cancer With Nutrition, (1994) Patrick Quillin, Ph.D., R.D., The Nutrition Times Press

Celebrating Life, (1995) Sylvia Dunnavant, USFI, Inc., Dallas, Texas.

Prescription for Nutritional Healing, (1997) James F. Balch, M.D. and Phyllis S. Balch, C.N.C., Avery Publishing, Garden City Park, N.Y.

The Breast Cancer Prevention Diet, (1998) Dr. Robert B.Arnot,
    Little, Brown & Co. Boston, N.Y., London.
Spontaneous Healing, (1995) by Andrew Weil, M.D., Knopf,
    Random House,.N.Y.
Why People Don't Heal and How They Can, Carol Myss, Ph.D.,
    Three Rivers Press, N.Y.

Guided Meditation Audio Cassettes

I make time to listen to guided meditations as often as
possible. The experience is relaxing, and research indicates that
the suggestions on these tapes reach the subconscious mind
and make a substantial impact. Some of the tapes I enjoy are:
Morning and Evening Meditation, Louise Hay
Cancer: Discovering Your Healing Power, Louise Hay
Getting Well, Dr. Carl Simonton
Peace, Alan Cohen and Steven Halpern
The Invitation to Healing, Beverly Hutchinson and
    Steven Halpern
How to Meditate, Lawrence LeShan

Natural Healing Agents and Preventative Measures

I recommend choosing a naturopath in addition to your
regular doctors. You can benefit from a specially designed diet.
Cancer patients are advised to follow a diet containing less than
thirty percent fat (my naturopath recommends no animal fat)
and to eat lots of fresh fruits and vegetables. Some vegetables,
such as carrots, broccoli, brussels sprouts, cabbage and cauli-
flower, are known to have cancer-fighting properties. Almonds
are thought by some health experts to be anti-carcinogenic.
Following are some of the supplements which I take in addition
to Tamoxifen. Do your own research and reach your own
conclusions as to whether this could be helpful to you.

Essiac

Essiac is a liquid herbal remedy which reportedly was

used with some degree of success by Rene Caisse, a Canadian nurse. The ingredients and further information may be obtained from Herbal Products Company in North Hollywood, California, (213) 877-3104.

Pau d'Arco

Available in tea or in tablet form, this supplement is derived from the inner bark of the Pau d'Arco tree and contains the active ingredient, lapachol. The substance has long been thought to have cancer-fighting qualities due to its antibacterial and cleansing properties. According to Patrick Quillin, Ph.D., R.D., the preliminary studies from the National Cancer Institute appear favorable.

Green Tea

Green tea is another natural substance which has been touted in the past few years for its effectiveness in preventing some types of cancer. Green tea contains the flavonoid catechin, a powerful antioxidant. The best-tasting brand I've discovered is Celestial Seasonings. I add a little honey for sweetness.

Co-Enzyme Q10

This enzyme is required in every cell of the body and reportedly has been used successfully in the treatment of some cancers when given in large doses. It is discussed at length in Dr. Patrick Quillin's book, *Beating Cancer With Nutrition* and in *Prescription for Nutritional Healing*, by James and Phyllis Balch. My naturopath recommended a daily dose of 100 milligrams, but do your own research.

Vitamin C

Linus Pauling was the pioneer in raising public awareness as to the value of Vitamin C in the treatment of cancer. On the recommendation of my naturopath, I take 10,000 milligrams daily. This high dosage may cause diarrhea. In the event of diarrhea, the dosage should be reduced immediately.

Good vs. Bad Fatty Acids

The types of fats ingested in the diet determine the strength of the signal from the estrogen receptor to the deoxyribonucleic acid, or DNA. DNA is the main component of chromosomes and is responsible for transferring the genetic characteristics. Cancer cells are marked by irregular DNA.

Omega-6 fatty acids send an extremely strong signal that is more likely to cause rapid cell growth. These undesirable fatty acids are found in such polyunsaturated fats as mayonnaise, many of the prepared salad dressings, corn oil, grape seed oil, peanut oil, primrose oil, safflower oil, sesame oil and, oddly enough, soybean oil.

Omega-3 fatty acids help prevent the risk of breast cancer by reducing the effect of the nasty omega-6 fatty acids. They send a weak signal from the estrogen receptors to the DNA. These good fatty acids are found in many fish oils and flaxseed. The recommended daily dosage is 10 grams per day. Again, do your own research.

Omega-9 fatty acids, found primarily in olive oil, are also beneficial in lowering the risk of breast cancer. I substitute olive oil for all cooking oil and salad oil as well as for butter or margarine in most recipes.

Flaxseed

Flaxseed is one of the most encouraging anti-carcinogenic foods on the market today. It contains two very important things: omega-3 (good) fatty acid and weak (good) plant estrogen.

The weak (plant) estrogen in flaxseed is also helpful in the fight against cancer due to its ability to latch onto the estrogen receptors and thus block the strong, harmful estrogen, such as estradiol.

The flaxseed must be ground in order to be absorbed properly. I add mine to a soy-protein drink and leave the blender running until it is well ground.

Soy

Soy is considered a plant estrogen. Many soy products contain a substance called genstein, which blocks strong estrogens from the receptors, decreasing the strength of the signal mentioned above. Soy also adds to the number of carriers that hook onto estrogen in the bloodstream and prevent it from attaching to receptors. Asian women have a much lower incidence of breast cancer than their American counterparts, and this is thought to be partly due to the large amounts of soy contained in the Asian diet. Soy oil and soy sauce do not have any beneficial effect in avoiding breast cancer. Soy oil should be avoided.

One recommended dosage is between 35 and 60 grams per day. If you have any questions about the wisdom of adding even weak estrogen to your system, consult a professional. I add soy-protein powder and flax seeds to orange juice and prepare a morning drink in my blender.

The Insulin Effect

Insulin, much like estrogen, contributes to the probability of breast cancer because of its tendency to exacerbate cell division. For that reason, a diet high in sugar should be avoided. Because North Americans tend to consume high quantities of sugar, cutting back on sugar can be a tough order. At the very least, we should avoid refined sugar and attempt to satisfy our craving for sweetness by filling up on fresh fruit, as recommended by the American Cancer Society, and adding a variety of fresh vegetables for balance.

Fiber

One way to counteract the sugar in our diet is to increase our intake of dietary fiber. By coating the lining of the colon, fiber slows the absorption of sugar and subsequently decreases the insulin level in the bloodstream. It also binds estrogen so that it is expelled properly from the body rather than being reabsorbed after digestion. Dr. Bob Arnot recommends at least 30 grams daily of dietary fiber. Two of the best cereals I've found are *Fiber One,* by General Mills, and *Kellogg's All Bran* with added fiber. Uncooked corn bran has one of the highest fiber contents of any grain. Beans are also a relatively good source.

I believe that many of these non-prescription formulas available can't hurt and may help. I want them as (possibly) added insurance. I take Tamoxifen, I show up for tests and appointments and I seek out anything which might raise my odds for survival.

The best and most complete books I have found dealing with diet and natural cancer treatments are *Breast Cancer, What You Should Know (But May Not Be Told),* Steven Austin, M.D. and Cathy Hitchcock, M.S.W., (1994, Prima Publishing, Rocklin, CA), *Beating Cancer With Nutrition*, Patrick Quillin, Ph.D., RD., 1994, (The Nutrition Times Press), Tulsa, OK., and *Prescription for Nutritional Healing*, James F. Balch, M.D. and Phyllis A. Balch, C.N.C. (1997, Avery Publishing Group) Garden City Park, N.Y.

Stress

An oncologist once pooh-poohed my opinion that stress increases our chances of cancer recurrence. He told me that we're not white rats. No, we're not. We're considerably more connected to our mental processes. Best medicine: staying as stress-free as humanly possible. We all have stress factors in our lives. Mine had to do with elder care. Some people have troubled teenagers, poor relationships and stressful jobs. Your body is trying to tell you something when you become ill. If you don't make some changes in your life, all of the procedures and drugs in the world will only be a temporary fix, no more effective than a bandage on a corpse.

Remove as many stress factors from your life as you can. Take time for yourself. Put your health needs first. You won't be any good to anyone dead. If I had arranged for Mama to live with Grace two years earlier, my time with her would have been more enjoyable, and she would have received better care. You can't do it all. Take time to get away... to read and meditate or listen to your favorite music. Exercise regularly. If you're healthy enough, run. Running gets the endorphins flowing. Walking is relaxing and helps to relieve stress. Join an aerobics class if you prefer to stay indoors.

Suggested Reading About Stress and the Immune System

Choices in Healing, (1992) Michael Lerner, The MIT Press.
Healing Words, (1993) Larry Dossey, Harper, San Francisco.
Head First, (1989) Norman Cousins, E.P. Dutton, N.Y.
Prescription for Nutritional Healing, (1997) James F. Balch,
    M.D. and Phyllis A. Balch, C.N.C. Avery Publishing Company.

Humor

In his book, *Anatomy of an Illness,* Norman Cousins espouses the value of humor in promoting healing. My sense of humor came to my rescue and helped me considerably as I worked through the anxiety and grief of breast cancer. Without laughter, I don't know where I would be today. A good belly laugh releases stress and restores a sense of well-being faster than anything I know of. The *Mary Tyler Moore Show* and *Taxi* have helped me on more than one occasion to chase off late-night anxiety attacks which threatened to keep me from getting a good sleep.

Outside Support

Most of us need someone who will listen. Internalizing our fear and anger can be damaging. If the idea of therapy doesn't appeal to you or for some reason is not available to you, seek out an appropriate support group or talk with a close friend. Good friends can often be more helpful than anyone.

A comprehensive list of regional support organizations can be found in Appendix C of *Dr. Susan Love's Breast Book.*

Activism

Becoming an activist to help erase breast cancer can be very empowering. Try to attend the *Race for the Cure* or or a similar event near you. In order to raise awareness and obtain funding for breast cancer research and education, talk to anyone who comes your way. Offer to speak with other women who have been recently diagnosed and don't know the ropes. Who knows? You might even save a life.

Love Your Body

Know that even a mastectomy can in no way rob you of your womanhood. You were never only your breasts. If they were extremely important to you, you can build new ones. And if you prefer not to do so, you are still that wonderful, grand, spiritual, feminine creation. Love her. Protect her. Nurture her. She's worth it.

8

Helpful Suggestions

Bathing with Drains

I solved this problem by hanging a belt around my neck. The drain is attached to the belt with a safety pin. Balancing drains on the side of the bathtub is risky. If the drain should slip off the edge of the tub, you won't like the knife-cutting pain it produces.

Bras

Unless you have very large breasts, you needn't pay $25 to $50 for an everyday bra. Buy a less expensive double-layered sports bra, available in most stores. I prefer a bra with the hooks in front. In order to place your prosthesis, make a two-inch cut in the inside layer vertically, directly in front of the seam which runs under the arm. Insert your prosthesis, and voila! It's as smooth as silk. There are no wrinkles, and it's perfect for form-fitting garments.

Undershirts

At first, I didn't think the following creation of mine would work, but it does. Buy a couple of thick undershirts or long tank tops that don't have a lot of stretch. Sew falsies into them for the days you'd just as soon go braless. You can use safety pins to anchor them to your waistband. (Baby safety pins work best.) This avoids the problem of having your chest move around as you turn from side to side. Falsies weigh less, they're comfortable, and they work well.

A Word to Family and Friends

Some people want to talk about their run-in with cancer, and others don't. We're all unique individuals and process experiences differently. If you don't know what to say, saying nothing is better than making some flip comment in an attempt to lighten the moment. I find any verbiage which trivializes my experience quite irritating and thoughtless. Breast cancer is no breeze even if one emerges with a slim chance of a recurrence. Facing one's mortality is a harrowing ordeal. The additional trauma of physical disfigurement, or the loss of hair brought on by chemotherapy is more salt poured into the wound. The best thing a friend or family member can do is to show how much you care and be understanding and patient with the occasional mood swings and withdrawal your loved one may display. It will all pass. Time does heal.

You can help by being an activist. I treasure my friends who attend the *Race for the Cure* and are involved in fund-raising for the cause. Between 1990 and 1992, activists such as the National Breast Cancer Coalition and Senator Tom Harkin were responsible for raising the annual breast cancer research budget from $89 million to $433 million. It truly *is* all about money and commitment. Think of the strides we've made in AIDS treatment in the last few years because of political activism. We can find a cure, and we will. We can make the words *breast cancer* an echo in the winds of yesterday. I hope you'll be a part of it.

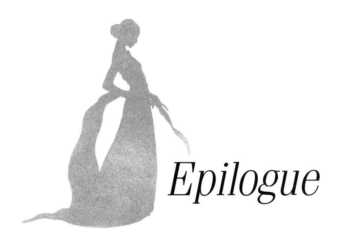

Epilogue

The past five years have no doubt been the most challenging ones of my life. After the tears and the questions, I have finally arrived at a point where I no longer feel the need to define my life by breast cancer. I'll remain an activist, but I shall never again permit myself to engage in the victim mentality or focus unnecessarily on my personal experience with the disease.

Since that cold day in November, I have celebrated my thirty-second wedding anniversary, watched my grandchildren grow, and made wonderful new friendships too numerous to count. I have breathed in deeply the sweet, clean scent of honeysuckle as I lie on my back looking up at the stars, and I have listened to Chopin and Massenet with my dog nestled gently in the crook of my arm.

My interlude with breast cancer has taught me many things. I believe I have come away stronger and more closely aligned with my spiritual side. Perhaps one of the most important things I have learned is that in order to be healed, we must be willing to change.

This may sound fairly simple, but most of us are pretty well settled into our comfort zones and the way we have done things for years, and we're quick to rationalize maintaining the status quo. Some of the changes may be drastic ones. In order to reduce the stress in our lives, we may have to leave our jobs and end toxic relationships. Most of us may need to overhaul our dietary patterns or get help to stop smoking or drinking. Difficult as these changes can be, they may be the only key to saving our lives. It was Bernie Siegel who said that many cancer patients would rather die than change, and from what I have observed in the last five years, I know that he is absolutely right.

The changes I've made in my life have given me a certain peace I never really had before. I look upon every day as a precious gift to be savored from the very depth of my spirit. Not one of us is guaranteed tomorrow; that is the lesson cancer has taught me. Though I would rather have learned that lesson in an easier, less life-threatening way, I will continue living in this place of gratitude, this place which God has allowed me to have for this very moment — and I hope, for many more to come.

A naturopath recently asked me whether I was "in remission." I guess that is one way of looking at it, but for as long as my tests come back without any signs of recurrence, I prefer to consider myself cured.

—Rachael Clearwater

To order additional copies of

Dreamwalk

Book $15 * Shipping/Handling $4
Call: BookPartners: 1-800-895-7323
Fax: 503-682-2057
e-mail: info@bookpartners.com

Or Call:
Voice: 503-231-5163
Fax: 503-234-4708
e-mail: clearskyreflections@worldnet.att.net

We accept Master Card * Visa * American Express

Ask us About Our Quantity Discounts

` ` ` ` ` ` ` `

How to Reach the Author:
e-mail: clearskyreflections@worldnet.att.net

BookPartners, Inc.
P.O.Box 922
Wilsonville, OR 97070